Past Papers

MRCOG Part One Multiple Choice Questions, 1997–2001

Royal College of Obstetricians and
Gynaecologists Examination Committee

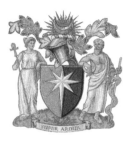

RCOG Press
September 2010

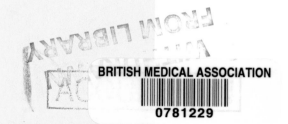

CAMBRIDGE
UNIVERSITY PRESS

University Printing House, Cambridge CB2 8BS, United Kingdom

Cambridge University Press is part of the University of Cambridge.

It furthers the University's mission by disseminating knowledge in the pursuit of education, learning and research at the highest international levels of excellence.

www.cambridge.org
Information on this title: www.cambridge.org/9781904752127

© 2004 The Royal College of Obstetricians and Gynaecologists

The use of registered names, trademarks, etc. in this publication does not imply, even in the absence of a specific statement, that such names are exempt from the relevant laws and regulations and therefore for general use.

While every effort has been made to ensure the accuracy of the information contained within this publication, the publisher can give no guarantee for information about drug dosage and application thereof contained in this book. In every individual case the respective user must check current indications and accuracy by consulting other pharmaceutical literature and following the guidelines laid down by the manufacturers of specific products and the relevant authorities in the country in which they are practising.

First published 2004
Reprinted 2010

A catalogue record for this publication is available from the British Library

ISBN 978-1-904-75212-7 Paperback

Cambridge University Press has no responsibility for the persistence or accuracy of URLs for external or third-party internet websites referred to in this publication, and does not guarantee that any content on such websites is, or will remain, accurate or appropriate.

Contents

Introduction

The Part One MRCOG examination is a test of basic science knowledge as applicable to obstetrics and gynaecology. While the format of the examination (two papers each of 300 multiple true/false questions) has remained unaltered over the past two decades, the syllabus and mix of questions has undergone considerable updating. The trainees of today will experience a massive influx of scientific knowledge in their practice over a lifetime, and the examination aims to equip trainees as best possible to understand, interpret and apply new knowledge properly.

With that principle in mind, the Part One Sub-committee of the RCOG has worked to introduce new and up-to-date questions into each examination. These are initially 'test' questions, which are marked and analysed by the Committee, but the marks do not count towards candidates' final score. This allows 'good', discriminating questions to be selected into the question bank and for 'poor' questions to be amended or discarded. Candidates' marks are therefore derived only from properly validated questions.

This publication is a landmark in the history of the Part One MRCOG. For the first time, candidates are able to study real questions and to self-assess their chances of passing the examination. The members of the Examination Committee hope that this information will encourage candidates to sit the examination when they are ready, while discouraging those who are too early in their cycle of learning.

The following series of questions are verbatim transcripts from the ten examinations set between 1997 and 2001, with test questions removed. The questions remain in the bank and may appear again in the future. We hope that they will be a useful aid to learning and we wish the candidates of the future every success.

Bill Ledger Chair, Part One MRCOG Sub-committee
(on behalf of the Examination Committee, RCOG)

March 1997
Paper 1

1. **Chromaffin cells**

A. are innervated by pre-ganglionic sympathetic nerve fibres.
B. are present in the adrenal cortex.
C. are derived from neuro-ectoderm.
D. can decarboxylate amino acids.
E. are present in coeliac ganglia.

2. **The internal pudendal artery**

A. leaves the pelvis through the lesser sciatic foramen.
B. lies on the medial wall of the ischiorectal fossa.
C. has a branch which pierces the perineal membrane.
D. gives rise to the middle rectal artery.
E. supplies the upper vagina.

3. **The pelvic splanchnic nerves**

A. are derived from the posterior rami of the sacral spinal nerves.
B. supply afferent fibres.
C. unite with branches of the sympathetic pelvic plexus.
D. supply the ascending colon with motor fibres.
E. supply the uterus with parasympathetic fibres.

4. **In the anterior abdominal wall**

A. rectus muscle is intersected transversely by three bands.
B. the posterior rectus sheath below the arcuate line consists of transversalis fascia only.
C. above the costal margin the posterior rectus sheath is deficient.
D. the superior epigastric artery arises from the internal thoracic artery.
E. the inferior epigastric artery arises from the femoral artery.

5. The rectum

A. is supplied in part by the inferior rectal artery.
B. is innervated by the inferior rectal nerve.
C. is lined by stratified squamous epithelium.
D. has its lymphatic drainage to the superficial inguinal nodes.
E. possesses a complete outer layer of longitudinal muscle.

6. The obturator nerve

A. emerges from the lateral border of psoas.
B. is formed from the posterior divisions of the second, third and fourth lumbar nerves.
C. passes lateral to the internal iliac vessels.
D. lies below the obturator artery in the obturator foramen.
E. is separated from the normally sited ovary only by the pelvic peritoneum.

7. In the cerebral cortex

A. the left visual field is represented in the right cerebral cortex.
B. the area directly concerned with movements of the face and hand is larger than that concerned with movements of the legs and trunk.
C. in most people, the left side is more concerned with speech than the right side.
D. pyramidal cells are present.
E. the blood supply is wholly from branches of the internal carotid arteries.

8. The cervix

A. consists chiefly of smooth muscle.
B. has a supravaginal part which is related anteriorly to the ureter.
C. has a supravaginal part which is covered with peritoneum, anteriorly.
D. has pain sensation carried by the pelvic splanchnic nerves.
E. is lined in its vaginal part by keratinised epithelium.

9. The right ureter lies in close relationship to the

A. bifurcation of the right common iliac artery.
B. infundibulopelvic ligament.
C. uterine artery.
D. inferior mesenteric artery.
E. parietal attachment of the sigmoid mesocolon.

10. The pelvic surface of the sacrum

A. gives origin to the piriformis muscle.
B. gives origin to the levator ani muscle.
C. is broader in the male than in the female.
D. transmits the dorsal rami of sacral nerves.
E. is in contact with the anal canal.

11. In the fetal circulation

A. the ductus venosus delivers blood directly into the superior vena cava.
B. the umbilical artery returns blood from the placenta.
C. the ductus arteriosus carries blood to the lungs.
D. blood returning from the lungs is 90% saturated with oxygen.
E. blood from the inferior vena cava is largely directed through the foramen ovale.

12. The ductus venosus

A. is part of the embryonic heart.
B. is a shunt preventing blood from passing to the fetal lungs.
C. gives rise to the ligamentum teres.
D. carries blood with a higher Po_2 than umbilical arterial blood.
E. is derived from the anterior cardinal vein.

13. The following structures take part in the formation of the anterior fontanelle in the fetal skull:

A. lambdoidal suture.
B. occipital suture.
C. sagittal suture.
D. glabella.
E. frontal suture.

14. Concerning the embryology of the urinary tract:

A. The detrusor has a mesodermal origin.
B. The urogenital sinus is derived from the cloaca.
C. The allantois gives origin to the lateral umbilical ligaments.
D. The metanephric ducts arise from the mesonephric ducts.
E. The mesonephric duct remnants form the epoophoron in the adult female.

15. The following tissues are paired with the appropriate primary germ cell layer of origin:

A. mammary duct epithelium : ectoderm.
B. epithelium of the tongue : mesoderm.
C. pineal gland : ectoderm.
D. ovarian stroma : mesoderm.
E. endometrium : mesoderm.

16. Adrenocorticotrophic hormone

A. production is governed by the hypothalamus.
B. production is maximal about midnight.
C. is present in the placenta.
D. is increased in the maternal plasma in pregnancy.
E. secretion is inhibited by glucocorticoids.

17. After the menopause,

A. the plasma concentration of follicle stimulating hormone increases.
B. the plasma progesterone concentration increases.
C. oestrone is the oestrogen found in highest concentration in the plasma.
D. the plasma testosterone concentration doubles.
E. the plasma prolactin concentration increases.

18. Successful lactation is

A. maintained by oestrogens.
B. maintained by progesterone.
C. initiated by a prolactin surge.
D. maintained by human placental lactogen.
E. inhibited by dopamine.

19. In a woman of reproductive age, serum concentrations of the following hormones exhibit a recognised pattern of diurnal variation:

A. progesterone.
B. melatonin.
C. cortisol.
D. oestrone.
E. follicle-stimulating hormone.

20. Serum concentrations of the following increase during pregnancy:

A. sex hormone-binding globulin.
B. prolactin.
C. total thyroxine.
D. follicle-stimulating hormone.
E. 17α-hydroxyprogesterone.

21. Luteinising hormone

A. is required for normal corpus luteum survival.
B. has a half-life in the circulation of 30 hours.
C. is released in pulses.
D. in the male stimulates testosterone production.
E. plasma concentrations are increased in postmenopausal women.

22. The release of catecholamines from the adrenal medulla increases

A. during sleep in healthy individuals.
B. when the nerves to the adrenal gland are stimulated.
C. following an increase in blood sugar.
D. immediately following a myocardial infarction.
E. during acute haemorrhage.

23. Prolactin

A. release is stimulated by thyrotrophin-releasing hormone.
B. plasma levels are raised in the first trimester of pregnancy.
C. release is increased by suckling.
D. may be produced by the decidua.
E. release is inhibited by metoclopramide.

24. Human chorionic gonadotrophin

A. is not produced by the decidua.
B. is biochemically indistinguishable from luteinising hormone.
C. is active if given to nonpregnant women.
D. production rises steadily throughout pregnancy.
E. has no influence upon the production of oestrogens by the placenta.

25. Human placental lactogen

A. concentration in maternal plasma is directly proportional to the functional mass of the placenta.
B. has a half-life in blood of less than 1 hour.
C. is a steroid hormone.
D. increases the mobilisation of maternal free fatty acids.
E. reaches the same concentration in fetal blood as in maternal blood at term.

26. The secretion of growth hormone

A. occurs in the hypothalamus.
B. ceases when the adult state is reached.
C. is decreased during stress.
D. is increased during fasting.
E. is increased with exercise.

27. Oxytocin

A. is released episodically.
B. causes decreased renal tubular reabsorption of water.
C. is responsible for milk ejection.
D. reduces intestinal peristalsis.
E. inhibits prolactin secretion.

28. Hirsutism in women is characteristically associated with

A. testicular feminisation.
B. Turner syndrome.
C. polycystic ovary syndrome.
D. arrhenoblastoma.
E. hypopituitarism.

29. Parathyroid hormone

A. decreases the renal excretion of phosphate.
B. increases calcium resorption from bone.
C. depresses pituitary activity.
D. concentrations in blood are raised when the calcium level falls.
E. increases renal tubular reabsorption of calcium.

30. Aldosterone

A. reduces sodium reabsorption in the proximal convoluted tubule.

B. reduces sodium absorption in the descending loop of Henle.
C. increases sodium absorption in the distal convoluted tubule.
D. increases potassium loss from the tubule.
E. increases sodium absorption in the collecting tubule.

31. Oestradiol-17β

A. is synthesised by aromatisation of testosterone.
B. vasodilates the uterine artery.
C. suppresses uterine activity by upregulating the oxytocin receptor.
D. promotes secondary sexual hair growth in females.
E. is thrombogenic.

32. The germination of tetanus spores in a wound is inhibited by

A. tissue trauma.
B. oxygen.
C. injection of anti-toxin.
D. injection of toxoid.
E. removal of devitalised tissue.

33. Proteolytic enzymes are secreted by the following organisms

A. *Neisseria meningitidis.*
B. *Salmonella typhi.*
C. *Streptococcus pyogenes.*
D. *Mycobacterium tuberculosis.*
E. *Clostridium perfringens (Welchii).*

34. Cytomegalovirus

A. is an adenovirus.
B. may be cultured readily in cell-free media.
C. is a cause of cerebral calcification.
D. causes haemolytic anaemia in the neonate.
E. may be transmitted in saliva.

35. The *Treponema pallidum* immobilisation test is positive in

A. yaws.
B. infectious mononucleosis.
C. malaria.
D. chancroid.
E. Lyme disease (borreliosis).

36. Leptospirosis

A. is caused by a Gram-negative coccobacillus.
B. is frequently transmitted to man from inanimate objects.
C. can result in a severe form of jaundice.
D. is a sexually transmitted disease.
E. is transmitted in pasteurised cow's milk.

37. Mycobacteria

A. are non-sporing.
B. are all acid-fast in their staining reaction.
C. are facultative anaerobes.
D. are responsible for leprosy.
E. are all pathogenic in humans.

38. The following disorders and organisms are correctly paired:

A. ophthalmia neonatorum : *Chlamydia trachomatis*.
B. chancroid : *Haemophilus ducreyii*.
C. sleeping sickness : *Leishmania donovani*.
D. ringworm : *Trichinella spiralis*.
E. non-specific uretiritis : *Toxoplasma gondii*.

39. The following organisms are Gram-positive:

A. *Mycoplasma hominis*.
B. *Staphylococcus aureus*.
C. *Clostridium perfringens*.
D. *Klebsiella pneumoniae*.
E. *Bacteroides fragilis*.

40. Concerning hepatitis B virus infection:

A. Vertical transmission does not occur.
B. Sexual transmission occurs.
C. Core antigenaemia indicates high infectivity.
D. Hepatocellular carcinoma is a recognised complication.
E. An effective vaccine is available.

41. The following antibiotics are usually effective against *Pseudomonas aeruginosa*:

A. cephradine.*
B. amoxycillin.
C. carbenicillin.
D. gentamicin.
E. trimethoprim.

42. Recognised unwanted effects of prostaglandin E include

A. water retention.
B. increased uterine contractility.
C. increased small bowel peristalsis.
D. flushing of the skin.
E. vomiting.

43. The following substances are sympathomimetic amines:

A. amphetamines.
B. ephedrine.
C. histamine.
D. isoprenaline.
E. chlorpromazine.

44. Subcutaneous atropine injection characteristically produces

A. an increase in heart rate.
B. an increase in salivation.
C. constriction of the pupil.
D. a hypnotic effect.
E. decreased bronchiolar secretion.

45. The following drugs have anti-cholinergic effects:

A. propantheline bromide.
B. carbachol.
C. distigmine bromide.
D. benzhexol.*
E. atropine.

---

* Registered international non-proprietary name is now cefradine; BNF 48, September 2004.

** Registered international non-proprietary name is now trihexyphenidyl; BNF 48, September 2004.

46. Treatment with morphine

A. causes respiratory depression.
B. increases gastric motility.
C. causes side effects, which may be reversed by naloxone.
D. increases the secretion of antidiuretic hormone.
E. causes pupillary dilatation.

47. Hypokalaemia may be caused by

A. bendrofluazide.*
B. digoxin.
C. spironolactone.
D. carbenoxolone.
E. amiloride.

48. Concerning heparins:

A. Heparin is synthesised in the lungs.
B. Antithrombin III is necessary for standard heparins to exert their anticoagulant effect.
C. Factor X is inhibited by low-molecular-weight heparins.
D. Low-molecular-weight heparins have a longer half-life than standard heparins.
E. Penicillins potentiate the action of low-molecular-weight heparins.

49. The following statistical statements are correct:

A. in the normal distribution, the value of the mode is 1.73 x that of the median.
B. in a distribution skew to the right, the mean lies to the left of the median.
C. in the series: 2;7;5;2;3;2;5;8, the mode is 2.
D. Student's t-test is designed to correct for skew distribution.
E. the Chi-squared test may be used when data are not normally distributed.

---

* Registered international non-proprietary name is now bendroflumethiazide; BNF 48, September 2004.

March 1997 Paper 2

1. The following changes in ventilation occur during pregnancy:

A. a decrease in respiratory rate.
B. a decrease in Pco_2.
C. a decrease in residual volume.
D. an increase in tidal volume.
E. an increase in Po_2.

2. The following are required for haemostatic clot formation:

A. conversion of prothrombin to thrombin.
B. platelet phospholipids.
C. active conversion of plasminogen to plasmin.
D. fibrin degradation products.
E. antithrombin.

3. Myometrial contractility

A. is calcium-dependent.
B. is associated with phosphorylation of myosin light chain.
C. is independent of cyclic adenosine monophosphate (CAMP).
D. is mediated by somatic nerves.
E. depends on myometrial gap junctions.

4. The following values fall within the normal range for the adult female bladder:

A. residual urine of 100 ml.
B. voiding volume of 250 ml.
C. bladder capacity of 900 ml.
D. intravesical pressure rise of less than 10 cm H_2O during early filling.
E. maximum urine flow rate of 60 ml per second.

5. The parenchymal cells of the liver

A. can convert fructose to glucose.
B. synthesise urea.
C. conjugate bilirubin.
D. excrete bromsulphthalein.
E. synthesise cholesterol.

6. In the testis,

A. maturation from spermatogonia to spermatozoa takes about 29 days.
B. Sertoli cells can mature into spermatids.
C. Leydig cells produce inhibin.
D. luteinising hormone inhibits the secretion of testosterone.
E. large quantities of fructose are present in seminal fluid.

7. Functions of the spleen in the healthy adult include

A. erythropoiesis.
B. destruction of erythrocytes.
C. formation of B lymphocytes.
D. phagocytosis of bacteria.
E. production of erythropoietin.

8. Neonatal jaundice may be caused by

A. congenital hypothyroidism.
B. phenylketonuria.
C. galactosaemia.
D. fructosaemia.
E. long-acting sulphonamides.

9. Concerning the vagus nerve:

A. When stimulated, it has little direct effect on the strength of the ventricular contraction.
B. It contains afferent nerve fibres.
C. Stimulation increases the heart rate.
D. It innervates the jejunum.
E. It is involved in the Hering–Breuer reflex.

10. In normal subjects the following increase ventilation:

A. a change in arterial Po_2 from 13.1 KPa (98 mmHg) to 8 KPa (60 mmHg).
B. a change in arterial pH from 7.36 to 7.48.
C. a change in arterial Pco_2 from 5.9 KPa (44 mmHg) to 8 KPa (60 mmHg)
D. administration of doxapram.
E. pregnancy.

11. The following statements relate to plasma proteins:

A. They create an oncotic pressure of 3.3 KPa (25 mmHg) across capillary walls.
B. They form a major part of the plasma cationic pool.
C. All are manufactured in the liver.
D. Albumin has a lower molecular weight than fibrinogen.
E. Fibrinogen is freely filtered at the glomerulus.

12. In a healthy, young, nonpregnant woman at rest

A. 80% of the body weight is water.
B. 75% of extracellular fluid is outside the blood vessels.
C. plasma volume is about 5 litres.
D. the pH of the plasma is about 7.25.
E. the plasma osmolality is about 400 mosmol/litre.

13. In the normal adult circulation

A. the pressure in the left ventricle during diastole is twice atmospheric pressure.
B. the aortic blood pressure during diastole is about two-thirds of that during systole.
C. resistance in peripheral blood vessels is inversely proportional to the fourth power of the vessel radius.
D. the arterioles are not subject to sympathetic stimulation except during exercise.
E. increased carotid sinus baroreceptor activity increases the heart rate.

14. The heart rate typically increases in response to

A. pain.
B. hypoxia.
C. ventilatory expiration.
D. increased intracranial pressure.
E. decreased baroreceptor activity.

15. In a healthy woman, renin

A. is secreted only by the kidney.
B. plasma concentration is greater in the pregnant than in the nonpregnant state.
C. plasma concentration is increased by diuretic therapy.
D. converts angiotensinogen into angiotensin II.
E. activity is blocked by captopril.

16. Concerning human parturition:

A. The number of oxytocin receptors in the myometrium increases before the onset of labour.
B. In the primigravida, cervical dilatation usually precedes cervical effacement.
C. The plasma oxytocin concentration increases at the onset of labour.
D. Oxytocin stimulates the synthesis of prostaglandins within the uterus.
E. Contraction of the maternal abdominal muscles is essential for spontaneous vaginal delivery.

17. Arterial plasma at 13 weeks of gestation in the normal pregnant woman

A. has a freezing point of 0.5°C.
B. has an osmolality of 190 mosmol/litre.
C. has a Pco_2 of 4 KPa (30 mmHg).
D. has a creatinine concentration of 200 µmol/litre (2.26 mg/ml).
E. has a sodium concentration of 140 mmol/litre (140 meq/litre).

18. Recognised effects of pregnancy include

A. transient impairment of glucose tolerance.
B. a raised glomerular filtration rate.
C. a raised plasma concentration of free tyrosine.
D. a reduced plasma concentration of alkaline phosphatase.
E. an increased secretion of prolactin.

19. In the small intestine the following substances are absorbed by active processes:

A. water.
B. sodium.
C. vitamin K.
D. amino acids.
E. chloride.

20. Collagen

A. has a double helical structure.
B. shows a regular banding pattern on electron microscopy.
C. is not formed normally in the absence of ascorbic acid.
D. is not found within basement membranes.
E. synthesis is inhibited by glucocorticoids.

21. White cell migration from blood vessels in areas of inflammation involves

A. cell migration occurring between endothelial cells.
B. a passive loss of fluid blood elements.
C. cell migration independent of endothelial cell motion.
D. initial emigration of polymorphonuclear neutrophils.
E. more polymorphs than monocytes after 2 days.

22. Carcinoma *in situ* in epithelium (intraepithelial neoplasia) is characterised by

A. increased mitotic activity.
B. loss of polarity.
C. increased adhesiveness to the underlying stroma.
D. pyknosis.
E. increased thickness of the epithelium.

23. The following provide conclusive evidence of pregnancy in uterine curettings:

A. decidua compacta.
B. Arias-Stella changes in endometrial glands.
C. spiral arterioles.
D. plasma cell infiltration.
E. chorionic villi.

24. In acute tubular necrosis of the kidney

A. the lesion is reversible.
B. the kidney is small.
C. 25% of deaths occur in the diuretic phase.
D. the distal convoluted tubules are mainly affected in mercury poisoning.
E. proteinaceous casts are found in the collecting ducts.

25. Complications of myocardial infarction include

A. fibrous pericarditis.
B. aortic aneurysm.
C. ventricular mural thrombi.
D. coronary atherosclerosis.
E. ventricular aneurysm.

26. In the pathogenesis of thrombosis

A. prostacyclin induces platelet aggregation
B. platelets synthesise thromboxane A_2.
C. thromboxane A_2 induces vasoconstriction.
D. contact with subendothelial collagen causes platelet aggregation.
E. thrombin inhibits platelet aggregation.

27. Characteristic features of Addisonian pernicious anaemia include

A. leucocytosis.
B. inheritance as an autosomal dominant trait.
C. a raised mean corpuscular haemoglobin concentration.
D. an increased incidence of gastric neoplasia.
E. an increased incidence of primary hypothyroidism.

28. Immunodeficiency states may be associated with

A. viral infection of T lymphocytes.
B. B cell lymphomas.
C. glucocorticoid administration.
D. haemolytic disease of the newborn.
E. untreated Hodgkin's lymphoma.

29. B lymphocytes

A. produce tumour necrosis factor.
B. produce complement.
C. produce antibodies.
D. contribute to delayed hypersensitivity.
E. produce IgE.

30. Antibodies

A. are proteins.
B. are formed in the fetus before 12 weeks of intrauterine life.
C. have an average molecular weight of around 10 000 daltons.
D. of the rhesus type are genetically transmitted.
E. are produced by the ribosomes of plasma cells.

31. Type III (immune complex-related) hypersensitivity is characterised by

A. damage localised to a particular cell type.
B. decreased vascular permeability.
C. microthrombus formation.
D. complement activation.
E. mediation by IgE antibodies.

32. The following disorders have an X-linked pattern of inheritance:

A. glucose-6-phosphate dehydrogenase deficiency.
B. Kleinfelter syndrome.
C. adrenogenital syndrome.
D. haemophilia B.
E. familial hypercholesterolaemia.

33. In the female,

A. only the X chromosome of maternal origin is active.
B. the Barr body is sex chromatin.
C. about 80% of polymorphonuclear leucocytes have a 'drumstick' of chromatin.
D. an extra X chromosome is associated with two Barr bodies.
E. an extra X chromosome is associated with below average intelligence.

34. In DNA,

A. a codon is a sequence of three bases.
B. all codons have an identified function.
C. there is a greater variety of amino acids than there are different codons.
D. replication can be initiated at several different points along a chromosome.
E. complementary pairing precedes messenger RNA synthesis.

35. The following genetic disorders are inherited as autosomal recessives:

A. Duchenne muscular dystrophy.
B. Huntingdon's chorea.
C. Tay–Sachs disease.
D. retinoblastoma.
E. achondroplasia.

36. In experimental conditions, ultrasound may produce biological effects on tissues by the following means:

A. acceleration of cell division.
B. heat generation.
C. cavitation.
D. duplication of chromosome numbers.
E. microstreaming.

37. Concerning radiation physics:

A. An electron has a greater mass than a proton.
B. A positron has the same charge as an electron.
C. A proton has a positive charge.
D. A neutron has almost the same mass as a proton.
E. The hydrogen nucleus is a neutron.

38. The conversion of glucose to lactic acid

A. occurs in a single enzymatic reaction.
B. is the only pathway for the synthesis of ATP in the red blood cell.
C. is a reversible process in skeletal muscle.
D. is inhibited by high cellular concentrations of ATP.
E. occurs in skeletal muscle when the availability of oxygen is limited.

39. Uric acid

A. is formed from the breakdown of purines.
B. is raised in serum during normal pregnancy.
C. is increased in serum during thiazide diuretic therapy.
D. is reabsorbed in the proximal renal tubule.
E. is excreted unchanged in the urine.

40. Adenine

A. is a pyrimidine base.
B. forms base pairs with thymine in RNA.
C. is synthesised attached to ribose phosphate.
D. can be converted directly to a nucleotide by the action of phosphoribosyl-transferase enzymes.
E. is degraded by a pathway which involves the enzyme xanthine oxidase.

41. Bilirubin

A. is a steroid.
B. is bound to albumin in the circulation.
C. conjugates iron.
D. is conjugated to glycerine.
E. facilitates absorption of fat from the gut.

42. Combined salt and water depletion is associated with

A. a high concentration of sodium in the urine.
B. a high urine specific gravity.
C. pre-renal uraemia.
D. a fall in the central venous pressure.
E. a high blood urea concentration.

43. Normal human seminal fluid

A. coagulates *in vitro*.
B. contains sucrose.
C. has a pH of 5.
D. may contain 15% of morphologically abnormal spermatozoa.
E. is predominantly produced within the testis.

44. Ethanol

A. consumed in excess stimulates fatty acid oxidation.
B. suppresses arginine vasopressin secretion.
C. promotes gluconeogenesis.
D. is oxidised to acetaldehyde.
E. is metabolised predominantly by the liver.

45. Glucocorticoids

A. promote hepatic gluconeogenesis.
B. suppress uptake of glucose by muscles.
C. promote protein breakdown.
D. promote fat breakdown.
E. increase glycolysis in adipose tissue.

46. Cholesterol

A. is an essential dietary requirement.
B. is present in the plasma membrane of all human cells.
C. cannot be synthesised by the liver.
D. is transported in the circulation bound to albumin.
E. is a precursor for the synthesis of steroid hormones.

47. Haemoglobin

A. has four porphyrin rings.
B. can carry four molecules of oxygen.
C. binds carbon monoxide more readily than oxygen.
D. is synthesised in mature erythrocytes.
E. contains two beta chains.

48. Fetal haemoglobin (HbF)

A. is not formed before 20 weeks of intrauterine life.
B. is more resistant than adult haemoglobin to denaturation by alkali.
C. in the fetus constitutes 80–90% of the haemoglobin at term.
D. represents less than 5% of total haemoglobin 8 weeks after birth.
E. is increased in adult patients with beta thalassaemia.

49. Fibrinogen

A. levels are usually low during pregnancy.
B. is a substrate for thrombin.
C. at elevated plasma levels causes a reduction in the erythrocyte sedimentation rate (ESR).
D. is synthesised in the liver.
E. is a Bence Jones' protein.

September 1997 Paper 1

1. The obturator artery

A. branches from the posterior trunk of the internal iliac artery.
B. passes through the greater sciatic foramen.
C. is crossed by the ureter.
D. supplies the hip joint.
E. may be replaced by a branch of the superior epigastric artery.

2. The spleen

A. has a notched posterior border.
B. lies in front of the costo-diaphragmatic recess.
C. is in contact with the body of the pancreas.
D. lies under the cover of the 9th to the 11th ribs.
E. is innervated from the renal plexus.

3. The following muscles are inserted into the perineal body

A. bulbospongiosus.
B. ischiocavernosus.
C. obturator internus.
D. sphincter ani externus.
E. transversus perinei superficialis.

4. The inferior vena cava

A. is formed at the level of the fifth lumbar vertebra.
B. commences posterior to the right external iliac artery.
C. receives the left ovarian vein.
D. receives the right renal vein.
E. pierces the central tendon of the diaphragm.

5. The adult female urethra

A. is 7 cm in length.

B.	is lined with columnar epithelium in its proximal half.
C.	has mucous glands in its distal third.
D.	passes through the perineal membrane.
E.	is surrounded by smooth muscle in its middle third.

### 6.	In the normal human pelvis

A.	the promontory of the sacrum is in the upper anterior border of the first sacral vertebra.
B.	the anterior surface of the sacrum has five paired foramina.
C.	the joint between the two pubic bones is a synovial joint.
D.	the acetabular fossa is wholly formed from parts of the pubic and ischial bones.
E.	the transverse diameter of the brim is greater than the antero-posterior diameter.

### 7.	The left ureter in the female

A.	develops from an outgrowth of the paramesonephric duct.
B.	when radiologically visualised, runs along the tips of the transverse processes of the lumbar vertebrae.
C.	is narrowed in calibre as it crosses the pelvic brim.
D.	runs medial to the ovary.
E.	lies anterior to the vagina as it enters the trigone of the bladder.

### 8.	Concerning the abdominal wall:

A.	The umbilicus is located in the territory of the L1 dermatome.
B.	The rectus abdominis muscle has attachments to the anterior wall of the rectus sheath.
C.	The left and right epigastric arteries anastomose.
D.	Distended veins radiating from the umbilicus are indicative of portal hypertension.
E.	Langer's lines run vertically over the lower abdomen.

### 9.	The pituitary gland

A.	lies below the diaphragma sellae.
B.	is developed from two primordia.
C.	communicates with the hypothalamus.
D.	lies inferior to the optic chiasma.
E.	is anterior to the sphenoidal sinus.

10. The obturator nerve

A. arises from segments L2, 3 and 4.
B. crosses the sacroiliac joint as it enters the pelvis.
C. innervates the obturator internus muscle.
D. is a lateral relation of the ovary.
E. innervates the knee joint.

11. Concerning cells:

A. Glycosylation takes place in the smooth endoplasmic reticulum.
B. Low density lipoproteins attach to cell membrane receptors.
C. Glycoproteins are present on the cytosol surface of the plasma membrane.
D. Centrioles are composed of tubulin.
E. Nuclear heterochromatin is genetically inactive.

12. The following are derived from the urogenital sinus:

A. the bladder trigone.
B. the ureters.
C. the female urethra.
D. greater vestibular glands.
E. paraurethral glands.

13. The following statements concerning the uterus are correct:

A. It is formed from the mesonephric ducts.
B. It has a lymphatic drainage in part to the inguinal glands.
C. The uterine artery passes below the ureter.
D. The uterine veins communicate with the vesical plexus of veins.
E. Pain sensation from the body of the uterus is carried by the pelvic splanchnic nerves.

14. In the fetal cardiovascular system

A. the heart arises from endoderm.
B. the heart is formed by fusion of endocardial tubes.
C. cardiac pulsation is present by the 30th day after fertilisation.
D. oxygenated blood is transferred to the left atrium through the foramen ovale.
E. the ductus arteriosus closes during the last 4 weeks of pregnancy.

15. Concerning growth hormone:

A. Plasma levels are reduced by glucose infusion.
B. Maternal plasma levels are directly related to fetal growth.
C. It is active on bone only until the epiphyses fuse.
D. Its secretion is controlled by the hypothalamus.
E. Increased activity produces a positive nitrogen balance.

16. Arginine vasopressin

A. reduces the glomerular filtration rate.
B. controls water loss in the proximal renal tubule.
C. is synthesised by the posterior pituitary gland.
D. is released in response to a rise in plasma osmolality.
E. is released in response to a fall in circulating plasma volume.

17. Parathyroid hormone

A. is a polypeptide.
B. increases bone resorption.
C. decreases phosphate excretion in the urine.
D. secretion is diminished by an increase in serum ionised calcium concentration.
E. decreases the formation of 1,25-dihydroxycholecalciferol.

18. Renin

A. is secreted by the zona glomerulose of the adrenal cortex.
B. is a proteolytic enzyme.
C. is secreted at an increased rate if the renal perfusion pressure falls.
D. acts upon circulating angiotensinogen.
E. is released in response to an increase in extracellular fluid volume.

19. Aldosterone secretion is increased

A. on standing.
B. following haemorrhage.
C. during pregnancy.
D. by hypocalcaemia.
E. on a low sodium diet.

20. Insulin secretion is stimulated by

A. gastrin.
B. noradrenaline (norepinephrine).

C. somatostatin.
D. glucagon.
E. arginine.

21. Concerning thyroid hormones:

A. Triiodothyronine is converted in the tissues to thyroxine.
B. The circulating concentration of thyroid binding globulin increases in pregnancy.
C. Triiodothyronine acts more rapidly than thyroxine.
D. Starvation causes plasma triiodothyronine concentrations to rise.
E. D-thyroxine is more active than L-thyroxine.

22. In the human testis

A. meiosis occurs between the early and late spermatid phases.
B. one spermatogonium always forms 8 spermatids.
C. the fluid in the seminiferous tubules contains a high concentration of protein.
D. the process of spermatogenesis takes 34 days.
E. inhibin is produced by primary spermatocytes.

23. Sex hormone-binding globulin

A. levels are increased in pregnancy.
B. is the main binding protein for progesterone.
C. levels are decreased during oestrogen therapy.
D. is the main binding protein for aldosterone.
E. has a greater affinity than albumin for testosterone.

24. Recognised features of congenital adrenal hyperplasia in the female are

A. acute hypotension.
B. enlargement of the clitoris.
C. abnormal karyotype.
D. hirsutism.
E. absent uterus.

25. Adrenal androgens

A. are synthesised in the zona glomerulosa of the adrenal cortex.
B. are secreted in excessive amounts in the presence of 11β-hydroxylase deficiency.
C. stimulate protein synthesis.

D.　consist mainly of testosterone.

E.　are secreted in increased amounts in response to a rise in adrenocorticotrophic hormone.

26.　During pregnancy, the uterine decidua synthesises

A.　human chorionic gonadotrophin.
B.　prostaglandin E_2.
C.　progesterone.
D.　prolactin.
E.　oxytocin.

27.　Calcitonin

A.　is synthesised in the parathyroid glands.
B.　is a decapeptide.
C.　secretion is increased at serum calcium levels below 1.5 mmol/1 (6.1 mg/l00 ml).
D.　inhibits bone resorption.
E.　increases renal tubular excretion of calcium.

28.　The following cell types are present in the human corpus luteum:

A.　endothelial cells.
B.　macrophages.
C.　pericytes.
D.　fibroblasts.
E.　granulosa cells.

29.　Concerning ovarian function:

A.　Progesterone is the major steroid of the developing follicle.
B.　Granulosa cells secrete oestradiol.
C.　Oestradiol is derived from androgen precursors.
D.　Insulin-like growth factor (IGF)-1 is not secreted by the ovary.
E.　Circulating inhibin concentrations are a marker of granulosa cell function.

30.　The following organisms are Gram-positive:

A.　*Streptococcus pneumoniae.*
B.　*Neisseria gonorrhoeae.*
C.　*Salmonella typhi.*
D.　*Lactobacillus.*
E.　*Pseudomonas aeruginosa.*

31. Toxic shock syndrome in women is

A. associated with the use of tampons.
B. due to a toxogenic strain of streptococcus.
C. a consequence of previous antibiotic therapy.
D. infrequently reported outside North America.
E. confined to sexually active women.

32. Concerning rubella:

A. It has an incubation period of 7–10 days.
B. Recurrent infection is a common cause of congenital malformation.
C. Specific antibodies occur within 14 days of infection.
D. Individuals are infectious before the appearance of the rash.
E. An attenuated live virus is used in immunisation.

33. Actinomyces israelii

A. is a rickettsia.
B. forms yellow granules in pus.
C. is a commensal in the mouth.
D. is a commensal in the vagina.
E. is usually resistant to penicillin.

34. Diseases caused by spirochaetes include

A. Weil's disease.
B. lymphogranuloma venereum.
C. pinta.
D. Vincent's angina.
E. bilharzia.

35. Mycobacterium tuberculosis

A. is the only mycobacterium which is acid-fast.
B. provokes humoral immunity only.
C. does not form spores.
D. is a motile bacillus.
E. produces endotoxins.

36. Candida albicans

A. is Gram-positive.
B. is a commensal in the bowel.
C. is sensitive to miconazole.

D. causes secondary infection after treatment with broad spectrum antibiotics.
E. is cultured on alkaline media.

37. The following antibiotics act on bacterial cell walls:

A. penicillin.
B. ceftazidime.
C. metronidazole.
D. clindamycin.
E. gentamicin.

38. Listeria monocytogenes

A. can grow at 6°C.
B. is a gut commensal.
C. is a Gram-negative bacillus.
D. infection is best treated with benzylpenicillin.
E. is a cause of septicaemia in neonates.

39. Metronidazole

A. is effective against *Giardia lamblia*.
B. is effective when administered per rectum.
C. should not be administered intravenously.
D. is usually effective against *Entamoeba histolytica*.
E. interferes with ethanol metabolism.

40. Gentamicin

A. is ineffective systemically when given by mouth.
B. is metabolised prior to excretion by the kidney.
C. may cause damage to the eighth cranial nerve.
D. is a bacteriostatic drug.
E. toxicity is potentiated by frusemide.*

41. The effectiveness of a combined oral contraceptive may be reduced by

A. bromocriptine.
B. phenytoin.
C. rifampicin.
D. ampicillin.
E. sodium valproate.

---

* Registered international non-proprietary name is now furosemide; BNF 48, September 2004.

42. The following agents are bronchodilators

A. salbutamol.
B. atenolol.
C. prostaglandin $F_{2\alpha}$.
D. morphine.
E. prednisolone.

43. Neostigmine in therapeutic doses

A. acts for several days.
B. inhibits hydrolysis of acetylcholine.
C. causes paralytic ileus.
D. reverses the action of carbachol.
E. relieves the effects of myasthenia.

44. Halothane produces

A. cardiac arrhythmias.
B. explosive mixtures with air.
C. liver damage if given repeatedly.
D. myometrial relaxation.
E. bronchial irritation.

45. The following substances increase the serum uric acid concentration:

A. colchicine.
B. chlorothiazide.*
C. allopurinol.
D. probenecid.
E. phenylbutazone.**

46. The therapeutic effect of the first drug is enhanced by the second drug

A. phenytoin : ethinyloestradiol.
B. bromocriptine : metoclopramide.
C. penicillin : probenecid.
D. ritodrine : dexamethasone.
E. warfarin : phenobarbitone.

---

* This drug has now been discontinued in the UK.
** Discontinued in the UK, September 2002.

47. In a sample of 1000 children, the birth weight was normally distributed with a mean of 3.5 kg and a standard deviation of 700 g:

A. 15 infants would be below the 5th centile for weight.
B. The standard error of the birth weight would be about 22 g.
C. The 95th centile for birth weight would be 4.2 kg.
D. No baby would weigh less than 1.4 kg.
E. The median birth weight would be about 3.5 kg.

48. In the statistical analysis of any group of numerical observations

A. the mean is always less than the mode.
B. the median value always lies at the mid-point of the range.
C. standard deviation is always greater than the standard error of the mean.
D. the standard error of the mean is independent of the total number of observations.
E. there are the same number of observations greater than and less than the median value.

49. In a randomised double-blind trial comparing a new drug with a placebo

A. the patients will be taking either of two active drugs.
B. patients can choose their method of treatment.
C. doctors prescribing treatment decide which patients take the new drug.
D. a large trial is more likely to give a statistically significant result than a small trial.
E. half of the patients will take the new drug.

50. In a trial of oral hypoglycaemic agents, 42 patients were given drug A and 38 drug B. Blood glucose concentrations were measured before and after a single dose of the drug. Drug B apparently caused a greater fall in blood glucose concentration ($P = 0.06$).

A. These results reach an accepted level of statistical significance.
B. Non-parametric statistical analysis should be used if data are not normally distributed.
C. In biological terms drugs A and B have been shown to be equally effective.
D. 6% more patients responded to drug A than drug B.
E. Unequal numbers in the two groups invalidate the trial.

September 1997 Paper 2

1. **Concerning pH:**

A. In blood, pH is regulated predominantly by bicarbonate.
B. The higher the pH, the higher the hydrogen ion concentration.
C. The pH of gastric acid is 5.5.
D. The pH of urine decreases after the ingestion of ammonium chloride.
E. The pH inside cells is higher than that in plasma.

2. **Concerning prostaglandins (PG):**

A. Arachidonic acid is the precursor for PG biosynthesis.
B. PG synthase (cyclooxygenase) catalyses arachidonic acid conversion to PG endoperoxides.
C. Nonsteroidal anti-inflammatory drugs inhibit PG dehydrogenase.
D. Mefenamic acid is a more potent inhibitor of PG synthesis than aspirin.
E. $PGF_{2\alpha}$ is excreted unchanged in urine.

3. **Peripheral concentrations of catecholamines increase**

A. during sleep.
B. when the nerves to the adrenal glands are stimulated.
C. when the blood sugar rises.
D. immediately following a myocardial infarction.
E. in the presence of a phaeochromocytoma.

4. **The rate of transfer of a substance into a cell by passive diffusion**

A. is unrelated to the concentration gradient.
B. is related to molecular size.
C. requires energy.
D. is different for stereo-isomers.
E. depends on carrier molecules in the cell wall.

5. Vitamin K

A. is synthesised by bacteria.
B. is stored in large quantities in the liver.
C. is necessary for the synthesis of factor VII.
D. is necessary for the synthesis of factor IX.
E. deficiency causes hypothrombinaemia.

6. Plasma concentrations of the following substances are typically raised in pregnancy:

A. caeruloplasmin.
B. albumin.
C. vitamin B_{12}.
D. urea.
E. pituitary gonadotrophins.

7. Potassium

A. is mainly intracellular.
B. plasma levels vary in proportion to intracellular levels.
C. plasma levels are decreased in Addison's disease.
D. plasma levels are increased in diabetic ketoacidosis.
E. deficiency occurs with prolonged vomiting.

8. In the neonate at birth

A. oxygenated haemoglobin is a less effective buffer than deoxygenated haemoglobin.
B. more than 50% of the circulating haemoglobin is haemoglobin F.
C. oxygen dissociation from haemoglobin is promoted by acidosis.
D. the total haemoglobin concentration is generally above 15 g/dl.
E. red blood cell 2,3-diphosphoglyceric acid is absent.

9. Triglycerides

A. contain glycerol combined with three identical fatty acids.
B. may accumulate in liver cells.
C. are present in intestinal cells.
D. are hydrolysed by pancreatic lipase.
E. are not present in chylomicrons.

10. Ribonucleic acid (RNA)

A. contains deoxyribose.
B. is composed of two nucleotide units.

C.   is the main constituent of human chromosomes.
D.   is the main constituent of ribosomes.
E.   is required during protein synthesis.

11. In one turn of the tricarboxylic acid cycle, three molecules of

A.   carbon dioxide (CO_2) are produced.
B.   reduced nicotinamide adenine dinucleotide (NADH) are produced.
C.   reduced dihydroflavine adenine dinucleotide ($FADH_2$) are produced.
D.   guanosine triphosphate (GTP) are produced.
E.   acetyl coenzyme A (acetyl CoA) are used.

12. Lactose

A.   is a non-reducing sugar.
B.   may be detected in the urine of a pregnant woman.
C.   is a major constituent of seminal fluid.
D.   is galactosyl glucose.
E.   is catabolised by the liver.

13. Concerning carbohydrates:

A.   Sucrose is a disaccharide of glucose and fructose.
B.   Cereal grains contain less than 40% starch.
C.   Cellulose is a fructose polysaccharide.
D.   A normal diet contains less than 60 g of carbohydrate daily.
E.   Dietary carbohydrate is oxidised in the body to carbon dioxide and
     water.

14. Muscle glycogen

A.   metabolism cannot yield free glucose.
B.   metabolism is independent of the enzyme phosphorylase.
C.   metabolism only generates ATP under aerobic conditions.
D.   is entirely intracellular.
E.   is released into the circulation in response to glucocorticoids.

15. The ultrasound energy used in a real-time machine for
     diagnostic imaging

A.   is pulsed.
B.   has a velocity measured in metres per second.
C.   has a velocity which is the same in all human tissues.
D.   has a frequency measured in decibels.
E.   is entirely dissipated within the tissues.

16. The natural decay of radioactive isotopes results in the emission of

A. alpha particles.
B. gamma rays.
C. neutron rays.
D. proton beams.
E. beta particles.

17. The following are inherited as autosomal recessive conditions:

A. tuberous sclerosis.
B. phenylketonuria.
C. ahondroplasia.
D. sickle cell anaemia.
E. Von Gierke's disease.

18. Genes on sex chromosomes are responsible for the inheritance of

A. glucose-6-phosphate dehydrogenase deficiency.
B. defective colour vision.
C. hairy ear rims.
D. homocystinuria.
E. Hurler syndrome.

19. The following genes and chromosomes are correctly paired:

A. HLA : chromosome 6.
B. clotting factor VIII : X chromosome.
C. glucose-6-phosphate dehydrogenase : X chromosome.
D. testis determining factor : X chromosome.
E. Xg blood group : chromosome 1.

20. In the human, a haploid number of chromosomes is found in

A. red blood cells.
B. blastocysts.
C. primary oocytes.
D. the first polar body.
E. spermatozoa.

21. **The following statements relate to familial diseases:**

A. Achondroplasia is a dominant trait.
B. Babies with Down syndrome usually have 46 chromosomes.
C. Congenital pyloric stenosis is commoner in babies of affected parents than in the general population.
D. All the daughters of a female carrier of red green colour blindness are themselves carriers.
E. Haemophilia occurs in all the sons of an affected father.

22. **Human immunoglobulin M (IgM)**

A. has a molecular weight of 150 000 Daltons.
B. contains J chains.
C. crosses the placenta readily.
D. fixes complement by the alternative pathway.
E. is a dimer in external secretions.

23. **Plasma cells**

A. are increased in myeloma.
B. are characteristic of acute infection.
C. are phagocytic.
D. synthesise immunoglobulins.
E. are derived from B lymphocytes.

24. **Antibodies play an important part in the development of**

A. phagocytosis.
B. the Mantoux response.
C. erythroblastosis fetalis.
D. hyperemesis gravidarum.
E. anaphylaxis.

25. **Osteoporosis is associated with**

A. an increase in uncalcified bone matrix (osteoid tissue).
B. prolonged oestrogen therapy.
C. a normal histological bone structure.
D. bone fractures.
E. irregularity of epiphyseal plates.

26. **Steps involved in the identification of restriction fragment length polymorphisms (RFLP) include**

A. Western blotting.
B. restriction enzyme digestion.
C. Southern blotting.
D. agarose gel electrophoresis.
E. thin layer chromatography.

27. **Features of disseminated intravascular coagulation include**

A. thrombocythaemia.
B. petechiae.
C. haemorrhage.
D. reduced circulating fibrin degradation products.
E. small vessel thrombosis.

28. **Chemical mediators concerned in the production of an inflammatory response include**

A. 5-hydroxytryptamine.
B. aldosterone.
C. glucocorticoids.
D. bradykinin.
E. leukotrienes.

29. **In sarcoidosis**

A. lesions are confined to the lung.
B. the Mantoux test is strongly positive.
C. caseation is not present.
D. the lesions contain giant cells.
E. the Kveim test is a useful adjunct to diagnosis.

30. **Adenocarcinoma is the commonest type of primary malignant tumour to occur in the**

A. bladder.
B. lung.
C. oesophagus.
D. fallopian tube.
E. testis.

31. The following tumours are correctly paired with likely causative agents:

A. angiocarcinoma of the liver : vinyl chloride.
B. carcinoma of the colon : dietary fibre.
C. hepatoma : aflatoxins.
D. carcinoma of the bronchus : coal dust.
E. carcinoma of the bladder : beta naphthylamine.

32. The parathyroid glands

A. originate from the pharyngeal cleft ectoderm.
B. secrete parathyroid hormone via the chief (principal) cells.
C. secrete calcitonin via the oxyphil cells.
D. may become hyperplastic in the presence of intestinal malabsorption.
E. may develop adenomas in association with islet cell tumours of the pancreas.

33. The concentration of urine

A. is due to passive reabsorption of water.
B. is completed in the loop of Henle.
C. occurs progressively along the proximal tubule.
D. is dependent upon arginine vasopressin.
E. is related to the osmolarity of the interstitial fluid of the renal medulla.

34. In the human neonate, compared with the adult

A. the liver has less ability to conjugate bilirubin.
B. the blood brain barrier is less permeable to bilirubin.
C. heat regulation is more efficient.
D. red blood cells have greater affinity for oxygen.
E. the haemoglobin concentration is greater.

35. Gastrointestinal absorption of

A. dietary glucose depends upon intact pancreatic function.
B. vitamin B_{12} requires gastric acid.
C. fats is accomplished by the transport of chylomicrons from the intestinal lumen.
D. iron may be reduced by vitamin C administration.
E. unhydrolised polysaccharides does not occur.

36. The menarche

A. usually follows an ovulatory cycle.
B. is preceded by the thelarche.
C. occurs earlier in girls below normal weight.
D. is preceded by the adrenarche.
E. is followed by the growth spurt.

37. Concerning platelets:

A. They are the only source of platelet-derived growth factor (PDGF).
B. Their life span is 90–120 days.
C. Average platelet count increases during pregnancy.
D. During aggregation, they release serotonin.
E. They contain platelet contractile protein (thrombasthenin).

38. Mast cells

A. normally form 3% of circulating leucocytes.
B. release histamine on degranulation.
C. contain heparin.
D. control melanin formation in the epidermis.
E. have a specific affinity for antibody of the IgA class.

39. Concerning the absorption of iron:

A. It occurs mainly in the ileum.
B. It normally represents 5–15% of the oral intake.
C. Its absorption is promoted by bile salts.
D. 10–15 mg dietary iron is required daily by a nonpregnant woman. between 20 and 40 years of age.
E. It occurs in the ferric form.

40. Characteristic features of Addisonian pernicious anaemia are

A. leucocytosis.
B. inheritance as an autosomal dominant trait.
C. a raised mean corpuscular haemoglobin concentration.
D. an increased incidence of gastric neoplasia.
E. an increased incidence of primary hypothyroidism.

41. The events in normal micturition in women include

A. contraction of the perineal muscles.
B. initial relaxation of the detrusor muscle.

C. a constant increase in intra-abdominal pressure.
D. no change in intravesical pressure.
E. Urinary flow of a maximum of 5 ml per second.

42. The following may occur in uncomplicated haemolytic jaundice

A. bilirubinuria.
B. high serum levels of conjugated bilirubin.
C. urobilinuria.
D. high serum levels of alkaline phosphatase.
E. reticulocytosis.

43. During the normal cell cycle

A. the principal phase of deoxyribonucleic acid (DNA) synthesis is G1.
B. a tetraploid quantity of DNA is present at the end of G2.
C. G2 is the post-mitotic resting phase.
D. cells are generally sensitive to anti-metabolites in the S phase.
E. the DNA is completely replicated several times.

44. In the renin–angiotensin system

A. oestrogen stimulates angiotensinogen production.
B. angiotensin II is converted to angiotensin I.
C. angiotensinogen is a globulin.
D. renin release is inhibited by sodium restriction.
E. renin may be produced by deciduas.

45. In the fetal circulation

A. most of the blood from the superior vena cava passes directly from the right to the left atrium.
B. the output of the right ventricle is greater than that of the left.
C. blood in the ascending aorta is more oxygenated than that in the descending aorta.
D. blood in the right ventricle is more oxygenated than blood in the left ventricle.
E. blood in the ductus arteriosus and the right atrium is equally oxygenated.

46. The adult oxygen–haemoglobin dissociation curve is shifted to the left by

A. low temperature.
B. low haemoglobin levels.

C. high altitude.
D. 2,3-diphosphoglyceride.
E. alkalosis.

47. The following factors increase ventilation in normal women

A. a rise in Pco_2 from 5.3 to 8.0 KPa (40–50 mmHg).
B. a fall in Po_2 from 13.1 to 11.7 KPa (98–88 mmHg).
C. pregnancy.
D. a fall in pH from 7.4 to 7.3.
E. taking a combined oral contraceptive pill.

48. Calcium in the serum of a healthy adult

A. constitutes 15% of total body calcium.
B. is not involved in the extrinsic system of blood coagulation.
C. has a concentration which is lowered by calcitonin.
D. has a concentration which normally falls after the menopause.
E. is approximately 90% protein-bound.

49. The stroke volume of the left ventricle

A. is equal to the blood volume in the ventricle at the end of diastole.
B. may be increased without increasing the end diastolic volume of the
    ventricle.
C. is directly related to the duration of the previous diastolic pause.
D. is consistently greater than that of the right ventricle.
E. is 20–30 ml in a resting man of average size in the supine position.

50. The following increase during normal pregnancy:

A. the basal metabolic rate.
B. serum cholesterol concentration.
C. fasting blood glucose concentration.
D. serum sodium concentration.
E. serum fibrinogen concentration.

March 1998 Paper 1

1. In the abdominal wall

A. the rectus abdominis muscle is attached to the crest of the pubis.
B. the posterior border of the external oblique muscle ends in the linea semilunaris.
C. the aponeurosis of the external oblique muscle takes part in the formation of the conjoint tendon.
D. the inferior epigastric artery is a branch of the internal iliac artery.
E. the conjoint tendon blends medially with the anterior layer of the rectus sheath.

2. The pelvic splanchnic nerves

A. contain parasympathetic fibres.
B. unite with branches of the sympathetic pelvic plexus.
C. are pre-ganglionic fibres.
D. supply the bladder sphincter with motor fibres.
E. supply the uterus with vasodilator fibres.

3. The vulva and perineum are supplied by the following nerves:

A. sciatic.
B. posterior cutaneous of thigh.
C. inferior rectal.
D. ilioinguinal.
E. obturator.

4. The adult spinal cord

A. commences at the foramen rotundum.
B. ends at the level of the upper lumbar vertebrae.
C. lies posterior to the spinal laminae.
D. is enclosed within a single layer of dura mater.
E. has a thoracic parasympathetic outflow.

5. The vaginal epithelium at puberty

A. thickens.
B. develops goblet cells.
C. forms cilia.
D. stores glycogen.
E. keratinises.

6. The urinary bladder

A. has an epithelium derived from endoderm.
B. has a venous plexus draining to the external iliac veins.
C. is situated in the abdomen of the young child.
D. is separated from the symphysis pubis by a fold of peritoneum.
E. has a blood supply from the inferior epigastric artery.

7. The following contribute to the boundaries of the ovarian fossa:

A. ureter.
B. external iliac vein.
C. internal iliac artery.
D. internal pudendal artery.
E. obliterated umbilical artery.

8. The following statements about the adrenal glands are correct:

A. They lie anterior to the diaphragm.
B. The left adrenal gland lies behind the pancreas.
C. Lymphatic drainage is to the superficial inguinal nodes.
D. The adrenal cortex contains chromaffin cells.
E. The adrenal medulla is derived from mesoderm.

9. The femoral ring

A. is lined by peritoneum.
B. is bounded medially by the lacunar ligament.
C. is bounded laterally by the femoral artery.
D. passes deep to the inguinal ligament.
E. is traversed by lymph vessels.

10. In the development of the heart

A. the primitive heart consists of five parts.
B. the septa are formed within 6 weeks of conception.
C. the septum secundum forms a complete partition in the atrial cavity.

D. obliteration of the right atrioventricular orifice is frequently associated with a ventricular septal defect.
E. anatomical closure of the ductus arteriosus occurs within 1 hour of birth.

11. **Concerning the development of the nervous system:**

A. The posterior neuropore closes before the anterior neuropore.
B. At 3 months of age, the spinal cord extends the length of the vertebral canal.
C. At birth, the spinal canal terminates at L3.
D. At birth, the dura mater extends as far as L3.
E. Myelin formation in the spinal cord is completed before birth.

12. **The urogenital sinus in the female gives rise to the following:**

A. ureter.
B. paraurethral glands.
C. Bartholin's glands.
D. urachus.
E. Gartner's duct.

13. **The mesoderm gives rise to**

A. striated muscle.
B. blood.
C. peritoneum.
D. transitional epithelium of the bladder.
E. ovarian stroma.

14. **Steroid hormones**

A. all contain 20 carbon atoms.
B. can be produced by structures of urogenital ridge origin.
C. are mostly activated in the liver.
D. are predominantly excreted unchanged in the urine.
E. mainly circulate unbound to carrier proteins.

15. **Human insulin**

A. is composed of two chains of amino acids.
B. differs from pig insulin by one amino acid.
C. facilitates glucose uptake by red blood cells.
D. increases protein synthesis in the liver.
E. increases triglyceride deposition in adipose tissue.

16. Thyroid hormones

A. increase oxygen consumption in most metabolically active tissues.
B. in the circulation are less than 90% bound to protein.
C. decrease the rate of absorption of carbohydrate from the gut.
D. increase circulating cholesterol concentrations.
E. are essential for skeletal maturation.

17. The interstitial (Leydig) cells of the testis

A. secrete seminal fluid.
B. are stimulated by luteinising hormone.
C. secrete androgen binding protein.
D. secrete fructose.
E. produce testosterone.

18. During the normal ovarian cycle

A. the principle oestrogen secreted is 17β-oestradiol.
B. the most potent oestrogen is oestriol.
C. oestrogen production is maximal by about the 8th day of the cycle.
D. oestrogens decrease the secretion of follicle-stimulating hormone.
E. oestrogens are synthesised primarily by the ovarian stroma.

19. Concerning sex hormones:

A. The ovary secretes androstenedione.
B. The ovary secretes testosterone.
C. The ovary secretes dihydrotestosterone.
D. Sex hormone-binding globulin (SHBG) concentrations are higher in women than in men.
E. Androgens bound to protein have high biological activity.

20. Progesterone

A. is synthesised by trophoblast.
B. increases myometrial activity.
C. is predominantly excreted in the urine as pregnanetriol.
D. binds to cortisol-binding globulin in the circulation.
E. is synthesised from cholesterol.

21. The hypothalamus is the site of synthesis of

A. oxytocin.
B. thyrotrophin-releasing hormone.
C. alpha melanocyte-stimulating hormone.

D. luteinising hormone.
E. gonadotrophin-releasing hormone.

22. During human lactation

A. oxytocin increases mammary duct pressure.
B. oestrogens promote the milk-producing effects of prolactin on the breast.
C. human placental lactogen is essential for milk synthesis.
D. prolactin stimulates gonadotrophin release.
E. suckling enhances prolactin release.

23. Follicle-stimulating hormone

A. binds to a receptor on the cell membrane.
B. promotes the expression of luteinising hormone receptors.
C. is responsible for the degeneration of the corpus luteum.
D. is a steroid hormone.
E. is synthesised in the hypothalamus.

24. Release of prolactin from the anterior pituitary gland is enhanced by

A. dopamine.
B. thyrotrophin-releasing hormone.
C. oestrogens.
D. chlorpromazine.
E. growth hormone.

25. Growth hormone

A. is a protein.
B. has a molecular weight of 2000 Daltons.
C. secretion is stimulated by hyperglycaemia.
D. has growth-promoting effects mediated through insulin-like growth factors.
E. is synthesised in the hypothalamus.

26. Arginine vasopressin

A. is produced in the hypothalamus.
B. is a polypeptide.
C. is structurally similar to prolactin.
D. controls water reabsorption by the kidney.
E. decreases glomerular filtration.

27. Hirsutism is associated with

A. testicular feminisation syndrome.
B. Turner syndrome.
C. Addison's disease.
D. Sertoli–Leydig cell tumours.
E. congenital adrenal hyperplasia.

28. Parathyroid hormone

A. increases bone resorption.
B. concentrations are increased in pregnancy.
C. reduces phosphate excretion in urine.
D. increases the formation of 1,25-dihydroxycholecalciferol.
E. stimulates osteoblasts.

29. Calcitonin

A. suppresses appetite.
B. is produced mainly in the thymus.
C. lowers plasma calcium concentrations.
D. secretion is inhibited by gastrin.
E. inhibits bone resorption.

30. Concerning viruses:

A. The core of every virus contains RNA.
B. They usually produce intracellular toxins causing cell death.
C. Antibodies are directed against capsular proteins.
D. They can only be grown in intact cells.
E. Interferons are synthetic antiviral substances.

31. The following are caused by herpes simplex virus:

A. acute gingivostomatitis.
B. cold sores.
C. cervical warts.
D. meningoencephalitis.
E. shingles.

32. Pertussis

A. is a viral infection.
B. is transmitted by droplet spread.
C. is associated with a lymphocytosis.

D. rarely occurs during the first year of life.
E. is effectively prevented by giving immunoglobulin.

33. *Pseudomonas aeruginosa*:

A. is non-motile.
B. is Gram-positive.
C. does not grow anaerobically.
D. ferments lactose.
E. produces pigment.

34. In septic shock

A. the causative organisms are invariably Gram-negative.
B. death is characterised by leucocytosis.
C. endotoxins are predominantly lipopolysaccharides.
D. antibiotic treatment may aggravate hypotension.
E. there may be associated disseminated intravascular coagulation.

35. *Candida albicans*

A. is a commensal organism in the bowel.
B. is Gram-negative.
C. forms pseudohyphae.
D. is sensitive to gentamicin.
E. reproduces by budding.

36. Features of congenital rubella include

A. excretion of virus by the neonate.
B. hepatomegaly.
C. excessive production of growth hormone.
D. cataract.
E. deafness.

37. Leptospirosis (Weil's disease)

A. produces a positive Wassermann reaction.
B. is associated with jaundice.
C. is transmitted to humans from rats.
D. infection is usually via the skin.
E. is a rickettsial infection.

38. Fluid retention may be caused by the administration of

A. spironolactone.
B. chlorothiazide.*
C. diethylstilboestrol.
D. carbenoxolone.
E. prednisolone.

39. The following have an antiemetic action:

A. hyoscine hydrobromide.
B. morphine sulphate.
C. chlorpropamide.
D. promethazine hydrochloride.
E. perphenazine.

40. Oestrogen therapy raises the plasma concentrations of

A. thyroxine-binding globulin.
B. free cortisol.
C. transferrin.
D. albumin.
E. folate.

41. The following compounds are predominantly progestogens:

A. buserelin.
B. dydrogesterone.
C. norethisterone.
D. 17α-hydroxyprogesterone.
E. androstenedione.

42. Clomifene citrate

A. is an anti-androgen.
B. does not stimulate ovulation directly.
C. can produce visual disturbances.
D. is generally prescribed throughout the proliferative phase of the menstrual cycle.
E. in the treatment of anovulation increases the risk of multiple pregnancy.

---

* This drug has now been discontinued in the UK.

43. The following statements describe the action of drugs on the myometrium:

A. Ergometrine stimulates sympathetic alpha receptors.
B. Indomethacin inhibits contractions by blocking prostaglandin receptors.
C. Prostaglandin E_1 is a stimulant or isolated uterine tissue *in vitro*.
D. Oxytocin requires ionised calcium as a co-factor.
E. Magnesium sulphate is a myometrial stimulant.

44. Sympathomimetic drugs in therapeutic doses

A. cause tachycardia.
B. cause hypotension.
C. cause a decrease in cardiac output.
D. cause arrhythmias in association with hydrocarbon anaesthetics.
E. are contraindicated in thyrotoxicosis.

45. Ventilation is increased due to stimulation of central receptors by

A. nikethamide.
B. hypoxia.
C. doxapram.
D. phenobarbitone.
E. salbutamol.

46. The following are cytotoxic alkylating agents:

A. cyclophosphamide.
B. mercaptopurine.
C. chlorambucil.
D. fluorouracil.
E. methotrexate.

47. The following statements are true:

A. Suxamethonium is a non-depolarising muscle relaxant.
B. Huxamethonium is a ganglion blocker.
C. Tubocurarine is reversed by neostigmine.
D. Streptomycin is absorbed from the gastrointestinal tract.
E. Thiopentone can be given intramuscularly.

48. If a distribution of results is markedly skewed to the left

A. the mean is the same as the 50th centile.
B. the same number of values lie on either side of the median.
C. the mode is equal to the median.
D. the Student's t test should be used to compare this distribution with another.
E. logarithmic transformation of the results will produce a distribution closer to the normal.

49. In a trial of a new therapeutic agent, the required sample size varies with the

A. level of statistical significance required.
B. level of acceptance of failing to discover a true effect.
C. type of statistical test to be employed.
D. magnitude of response expected.
E. experience of the investigator.

50. For international comparisons, the World Health Organization recommends that calculation of the perinatal mortality rate should

A. include all fetuses and infants weighing 1000 g or more.
B. include all fetuses and infants of a gestational age of more than 20 weeks.
C. include all fetuses and infants with a crown rump length of more than 35 cm.
D. be expressed as deaths per thousand live births.
E. include all deaths occurring in the first month of life.

March 1998 Paper 2

1. The oxidation of pyruvate to carbon dioxide

A. occurs exclusively in mitochondria.
B. can occur under anaerobic conditions.
C. involves intermediates that are also involved in amino acid catabolism.
D. is regulated by the concentration of acetyl coenzyme A in the cell.
E. is impaired in thiamine deficiency states.

2. Uric acid

A. is formed from the breakdown of purines.
B. serum concentrations are raised during normal pregnancy.
C. serum concentrations are increased during thiazide diuretic therapy.
D. is reabsorbed in the proximal renal tubule.
E. is excreted unchanged in the urine.

3. Creatinine

A. is filtered out by the glomerulus.
B. is reabsorbed significantly by the proximal tubules.
C. plasma concentration increases after protein ingestion.
D. has a plasma clearance rate equivalent to renal plasma flow.
E. plasma concentration increases during the first trimester of pregnancy.

4. Plasma albumin binds the following

A. free fatty acids.
B. triglycerides.
C. oestradiol.
D. bilirubin.
E. iron ions.

5. In the digestive system

A. polysaccharides are broken down mainly in the stomach.
B. one molecule of sucrose forms two molecules of glucose.
C. glucose transport into the cell depends upon the active transport of sodium ions.
D. fructose is mainly absorbed by simple diffusion.
E. lactase activity increases during childhood.

6. Methionine

A. is an essential amino acid.
B. is a sulphur-containing amino acid.
C. cannot be converted to cystine by the fetal liver.
D. cannot cross the placenta.
E. is reabsorbed in the proximal convoluted tubule in the kidneys.

7. Tetrahydrofolic acid

A. is involved in purine synthesis.
B. is a precursor of folic acid.
C. is a coenzyme in amino acid synthesis.
D. catalyses the conversion of glucose to glucose-6-phosphate.
E. activity is inhibited by methotrexate.

8. Deficiency of the following substances and diseases are correctly matched:

A. thiamine : pellagra.
B. cyanocobalamin : microcytic anaemia.
C. niacin : beriberi.
D. folates : sprue.
E. ascorbic acid : night blindness.

9. Fetal pulmonary surfactant

A. contains less than 10% lipid.
B. can be detected in amniotic fluid.
C. contains phosphatidylglycerol.
D. is predominantly dipalmitol-phosphatidylcholine.
E. is more than 40% albumin.

10. Standard bicarbonate in blood

A. is usually more than 30 mmol/l.
B. is increased with chronic carbon dioxide retention.

C.   is decreased with persistent vomiting.
D.   is decreased in renal failure.
E.   is decreased in severe diarrhoea.

11. Hyperkalaemia occurs in association with

A.   chronic diarrhoea.
B.   renal tubular acidosis.
C.   hypoparathyroidism.
D.   hormone-secreting tumours of the bronchus.
E.   primary hyperaldosteronism.

12. DNA

A.   contains no cytosine.
B.   has a background of ribose.
C.   is usually single stranded in mammalian cells.
D.   is cleaved by restriction enzymes.
E.   is irreversibly damaged in vitro by heating to 75°C.

13. Pancreatic glucagon

A.   is secreted by the beta cells.
B.   is a steroid hormone.
C.   secretion is inversely proportional to the blood glucose
     concentration.
D.   increases the breakdown of liver glycogen.
E.   increases the breakdown of triglycerides.

14. Biochemical abnormalities associated with diabetes mellitus include

A.   increased breakdown of protein.
B.   decreased plasma levels of free fatty acids.
C.   increased serum cholesterol concentrations.
D.   decreased glycosylation of haemoglobin.
E.   a decrease in the plasma concentration of low density lipoproteins.

15. The following substances are normally synthesised in the liver

A.   glucagon.
B.   vitamin A.
C.   cholesterol.
D.   immunoglobulins.
E.   prothrombin.

16. Radiation damage to tissue

A. is greatest in tissue with a high mitotic index.
B. is enhanced in the presence of a reduced oxygen tension.
C. may cause a non-specific inflammatory response.
D. does not cause neoplasia.
E. may cause chromosomal non-disjunction.

17. Mitochondrial DNA

A. is located in the nucleus.
B. inheritance is patrilineal.
C. is present in two copies per cell.
D. mutation causes cystic fibrosis.
E. is involved in the control of oxidative phosphorylation.

18. Concerning the genetic control of protein synthesis:

A. Mature messenger RNA contains introns.
B. A codon has 3-base sequences.
C. Each amino acid has a single codon.
D. Transfer RNA has anticodon recognition sites.
E. Each transfer RNA carries a specific amino acid.

19. When a man has haemophilia

A. 50% of his daughters would not expect to be carriers.
B. 25% of his sons would be expected to be affected.
C. good medical control of his blood deficiency reduces the risk of the condition in his children.
D. his newborn child is likely to require an urgent blood transfusion.
E. his sister has a 50% probability of being a carrier.

20. The human major histocompatibility complex (MHC)

A. resides on chromosome 11.
B. is composed of human leucocyte antigen (HLA) genes.
C. codes for three classes of antigens.
D. will be identical in dizygotic twins.
E. codes for blood group antigens.

21. Type-III hypersensitivity

A. is mediated by specifically-sensitised T lymphocytes.
B. causes myasthenia gravis.

C.   occurs in systemic lupus erythematosus.
D.   is a recognised cause of glomerulonephritis.
E.   may cause allergic asthma.

22.   The following cells are correctly paired with their products:

A.   endothelial cell : factor VIII related antigen.
B.   plasma cell : IgG.
C.   salivary gland epithelial cell : amylase.
D.   mast cell : IgA.
E.   decidual stromal cell : prolactin.

23.   The following are recognised functions of T lymphocytes:

A.   antibody production.
B.   cell-mediated immunity.
C.   immune suppression.
D.   phagocytosis.
E.   lymphokine production.

24.   The development of tissue necrosis

A.   can be identified by light microscopy within 1 hour of myocardial infarction.
B.   is recognised by the presence of karyorrhexis.
C.   is of colliquative type in the kidney.
D.   occurs in tertiary syphilis.
E.   is associated with rupture of lysosomes.

25.   The following statements relate to embryonic tumours:

A.   An ovarian teratoma is usually malignant.
B.   A nephroblastoma may be benign.
C.   A neuroblastoma can arise in the adrenal medulla.
D.   A hamartoma is usually malignant.
E.   Choriocarcinoma may arise in a teratoma.

26.   The parathyroid glands

A.   originate from the pharyngeal cleft ectoderm.
B.   secrete parathyroid hormone via the chief cells.
C.   secrete calcitonin via the oxyphil cells.
D.   may become hyperplastic in the presence of intestinal malabsorption.
E.   may develop adenomas in association with islet cell tumours of the pancreas.

27. The following conditions may lead to hydronephrosis:

A. mercury poisoning.
B. cervical carcinoma.
C. renal calculi.
D. renal vein thrombosis.
E. posterior urethral valves.

28. The following are X-linked disorders:

A. myotonic dystrophy.
B. Duchenne muscular dystrophy.
C. haemophilia A.
D. Huntington's disease.
E. fragile X syndrome.

29. A metaplastic process is involved in the histogenesis of the following tumours:

A. squamous cell carcinoma of the vulva.
B. squamous cell carcinoma of the bronchus.
C. scirrhous carcinoma of the breast.
D. squamous cell carcinoma of the cervix.
E. adenocarcinoma of the oesophagus.

30. Amyloid deposition is part of the pathological process in the following diseases:

A. medullary carcinoma of the thyroid.
B. plasmacytoma.
C. diabetes mellitus.
D. chronic pyelonephritis.
E. bronchial asthma.

31. Metastases to lymph nodes are commonly associated with

A. fibrosarcoma.
B. malignant melanoma.
C. medulloblastoma.
D. seminoma of the testis.
E. basal cell carcinoma of the skin.

32. Adenocarcinoma of the large bowel

A. most commonly originates in the ascending colon.
B. may develop as a single polyp.

C.   may show signet ring features histologically.
D.   characteristically metastasises to the liver before the lymph nodes.
E.   is a recognised complication of long-standing ulcerative colitis.

33.   Rickets is characterised by the following:

A.   mineralisation of the periosteum.
B.   deposition of uncalcified osteoid.
C.   abnormal osteoblastic activity.
D.   increased capillary fragility.
E.   overgrowth of cartilage.

34.   The following substances are correctly paired with their site of release:

A.   acetylcholine : postganglionic parasympathetic nerve endings.
B.   noradrenaline : pre-ganglionic sympathetic nerve endings.
C.   dopamine : hypothalamus.
D.   oxytocin : posterior pituitary.
E.   gonadotrophin releasing hormone : anterior pituitary.

35.   2,3-diphosphoglycerate

A.   is present at higher concentrations in maternal erythrocytes than fetal erythrocytes.
B.   binds to HbA more avidly than to HbF.
C.   increases the affinity of haemoglobin for oxygen.
D.   is a phospholipid.
E.   is synthesised by the pentose phosphate pathway.

36.   Platelets

A.   are approximately 50 micrometers in diameter.
B.   contain myosin.
C.   release a growth factor.
D.   are formed from myeloblasts.
E.   are prevented from aggregating by thromboxane A_2.

37.   In uncomplicated homozygous beta thalassaemia there is

A.   hypochromasia.
B.   a reduction in haemoglobin A_2.
C.   an increase in haemoglobin F.
D.   no depletion of iron stores.
E.   the presence of megaloblasts in bone marrow.

38. In the nephron, sodium

A. is mainly reabsorbed in the proximal convoluted tubule.
B. reabsorption increases in normal pregnancy.
C. may be reabsorbed in exchange for hydrogen ion.
D. reabsorption is increased by spironolactone.
E. reabsorption is increased by atrial natriuretic peptide.

39. Concerning normal urinary bladder function:

A. The bladder normally fills at a rate of 20 ml per minute.
B. During early filling there is minimal rise in intravesical pressure.
C. A significant increase in intravesical pressure occurs when the bladder contains 100 ml of urine.
D. The sensation of bladder filling is transmitted by the pelvic splanchnic nerves.
E. Micturition is initiated by contraction of the trigone.

40. The conjugation of bilirubin

A. takes place in hepatocytes.
B. is catalysed by UDP glucuronyl transferase.
C. is inhibited by phenobarbitone.
D. renders it water soluble.
E. is impaired in acute biliary obstruction.

41. Bradykinin

A. increases capillary permeability.
B. is a small polypeptide.
C. is formed by the action of kallikrein.
D. is predominantly inactivated in the liver.
E. is metabolised to kininogen.

42. 'Physiological' jaundice of the newborn

A. is present on the first day of life.
B. is due to ABO incompatibility.
C. is associated with a raised serum concentration of glutamic pyruvic transaminase.
D. may be due to relative glucuronyl transferase deficiency.
E. is associated with a raised level of unconjugated bilirubin.

43. Carbon dioxide

A. is produced in the body primarily from the decarboxylation of ketoacids.
B. makes up about 1% of the normal atmosphere.
C. occurs in normal arterial blood at a partial pressure of 8 KPa (60 mmHg).
D. is more water soluble than oxygen.
E. crosses the placenta at half the rate of oxygen.

44. The stimulation of adrenergic alpha receptors

A. does not occur with noradrenaline.
B. in the blood vessels of the skin leads to vasoconstriction.
C. in the gastrointestinal sphincter muscles leads to relaxation.
D. in the iris leads to constriction of the pupil.
E. in the blood vessels of the kidney leads to vasodilatation.

45. The following statements relate to lung function in normal pregnancy:

A. Vital capacity is increased by about 50%.
B. Tidal volume is increased.
C. The subcostal angle increases.
D. The residual volume is reduced.
E. The respiratory rate is increased.

46. Interstitial fluid in a healthy adult

A. contains virtually no albumin.
B. makes up about 70% of the total body weight.
C. is reabsorbed into the capillaries by simple diffusion.
D. will increase in response to histamine release.
E. accumulates in dependent parts of the body.

47. The erythrocyte sedimentation rate (ESR) is increased

A. following the infusion of high molecular weight dextran.
B. when plasma fibrinogen concentrations increase.
C. in men compared with women.
D. in old age.
E. in polycythaemia rubra vera.

48. Concerning blood pressure regulation:

A. Adrenaline acts primarily upon the vasomotor centre.
B. Prostacyclin lowers blood pressure.
C. Angiotensinogen is inactive without modification.
D. Bradykinin increases blood pressure.
E. Serotonin is vasodilatory.

49. In normal pregnancy, uterine blood flow

A. is about 50 ml/minute at term.
B. within the choriodecidual space is maintained throughout the cardiac cycle.
C. is reduced by prostacyclin.
D. is increased during uterine contractions.
E. represents about 10% of the cardiac output by the end of the first trimester.

50. During normal pregnancy

A. arterial Pco_2 decreases.
B. the blood hydrogen ion concentration decreases.
C. plasma bicarbonate concentrations decrease.
D. urine pH falls.
E. lactic acid production is increased.

September 1998 Paper 1

1. The pineal gland

A. is situated at the anterior end of the third ventricle.
B. is innervated by the parasympathetic nervous system.
C. produces melatonin.
D. may be calcified in the adult.
E. is most active during daylight.

2. The anal canal

A. has an upper part which is innervated by the inferior hypogastric plexus.
B. has a lower part which is supplied by the superior rectal artery.
C. drains lymph to the superficial inguinal nodes from its upper part.
D. has its internal sphincter innervated by the inferior rectal nerve.
E. has a superficial part of its external sphincter attached to the coccyx.

3. The pudendal nerve

A. arises from the posterior rami of S2, 3 and 4.
B. leaves the pelvis through the lesser sciatic foramen.
C. crosses the ischial spine on the lateral side of the internal pudendal artery.
D. supplies the levator ani.
E. supplies the clitoris.

4. The pelvic splanchnic nerves

A. are derived from the posterior rami of the sacral spinal nerves.
B. supply afferent fibres.
C. unite with branches of the sympathetic pelvic plexus.
D. supply the ascending colon with motor fibres.
E. supply the uterus with parasympathetic fibres.

5. **In the vulva**

A. blood is supplied by the internal pudendal artery.
B. the anterior parts of the labia majora are innervated by the obturator nerves.
C. the posterior parts of the labia majora are innervated by the genitofemoral nerves.
D. the lesser vestibular glands lie deep to the bulb of the vestibule.
E. the round ligaments of the uterus terminate in the labia minora.

6. **In the ovary**

A. primordial germ cells are formed.
B. primary oocytes have completed the first mitotic division by birth.
C. the majority of primary oocytes become atretic by puberty.
D. fewer than ten follicles start the process of antrum formation in each ovarian cycle.
E. the second polar body is formed at ovulation.

7. **In the human testis**

A. secondary spermatocytes contain 23 chromosomes.
B. one secondary spermatocyte forms two spermatids.
C. the seminiferous tubules contain motile spermatozoa.
D. the process of spermatogenesis takes 34 days.
E. inhibin is produced by primary spermatocytes.

8. **In the female, the ureter**

A. is separated from the sacroiliac joint by the bifurcation of the common iliac artery.
B. descends in front of the internal iliac artery.
C. passes behind the sigmoid mesocolon on the right side.
D. lies 5 cm lateral to the lateral vaginal fornix.
E. crosses superior to the uterine artery in the broad ligament.

9. **Concerning the urinary bladder:**

A. Its motor innervation is predominantly derived from the first sacral spinal segment.
B. In the empty adult bladder the ureteric orifices are about 2.5 cm apart.
C. The trigonal epithelial cells are mainly columnar.
D. Nerve plexuses in the detrusor contain acetylcholinesterase.
E. Its arterial supply is derived from the posterior trunk of the internal iliac artery.

10. The following structures pass beneath the inguinal ligament:

A.   ilioinguinal nerve.
B.   femoral artery.
C.   femoral branch of the genitofemoral nerve.
D.   superficial epigastric artery.
E.   lateral femoral cutaneous nerve.

11.   The umbilical cord

A.   contains mid-gut during embryonic development.
B.   is covered by amnion.
C.   consists chiefly of fetal endodermal cells.
D.   contains two veins and an artery.
E.   is approximately 50 cm long at term.

12.   The fetal testes

A.   are morphologically distinguishable 4 weeks after conception.
B.   contain cells which have migrated from the wall of the yolk sac.
C.   are usually intra-abdominal 12 weeks after conception.
D.   are necessary for the persistence of the mesonephric (Wolffian) ducts.
E.   secrete androgens.

13.   Concerning embryological development:

A.   The amnion has an endodermal origin.
B.   Uterine epithelium is developed from the paramesonephric ducts.
C.   The hymen develops at the junction of the synovaginal bulbs and the urogenital sinus.
D.   The round ligament of the uterus is derived from the gubernaculum.
E.   The adrenal cortex is derived from neural crest cells.

14.   Glucagon promotes

A.   hepatic gluconeogenesis.
B.   glucose uptake by muscle.
C.   glycogen synthesis by muscle.
D.   breakdown of protein.
E.   synthesis of fat.

15. Insulin secretion

A. is partly controlled by the direct action of blood glucose upon the pancreas.
B. affects the rate of entry of glucose into the beta cells of the pancreatic islets.
C. is stimulated by adrenaline.
D. is stimulated by arginine.
E. is stimulated more effectively by glucose administered intravenously than by glucose administered orally.

16. Concerning thyroid function:

A. Oestrogen increases the production of thyroxine-binding globulin.
B. More than 98% of circulating thyroxine is bound to thyroxine-binding globulin.
C. Thyrotrophin-releasing hormone is a decapeptide.
D. Thyroid-stimulating hormone levels are increased in primary hypothyroidism.
E. Thyroid-stimulating hormone is a glycoprotein.

17. Testosterone

A. is produced only in the gonads.
B. is mainly excreted unchanged in the urine.
C. stimulates secretion of luteinising hormone.
D. circulates in plasma mainly in the free form.
E. stimulates growth of the prostate gland.

18. In congenital adrenal cortical hyperplasia

A. the commonest deficiency is C18 hydroxylase.
B. plasma cortisol concentration is raised.
C. urinary excretion of 17-oxysteroids is elevated.
D. dexamethasone will suppress the urinary excretion of 17-oxysteroids.
E. there are no virilising effects.

19. Therapeutic indications for the use of synthetic progestagens include

A. induction of abortion.
B. contraception.
C. metastatic endometrial carcinoma.
D. suppression of lactation.
E. endometriosis.

20. In hypopituitarism

A. clinical features of deficiency are usually absent until about 70% of the gland has been destroyed.
B. thyroid-stimulating hormone is usually the first hormone to be affected.
C. aldosterone secretion is normal.
D. orthostatic hypotension is common.
E. hypoglycaemia occurs on fasting.

21. The following statements concerning the formation of hormones are correct:

A. ACTH is derived from pro-opiomelanocortin.
B. Oestrogens are derived from androgens.
C. Prolactin is derived from dopamine.
D. Melatonin is derived from serotonin.
E. Angiotensin II is derived from rennin.

22. Pulsatile secretion of pituitary luteinising hormone

A. increases in amplitude during puberty.
B. occurs in the first year of life.
C. ceases at the menopause.
D. is controlled by continuous secretion of gonadotrophin-releasing hormone.
E. is modified by the level of circulating oestrogen.

23. Adrenaline (epinephrine)

A. stimulates myometrial contractions.
B. exerts its action by alpha receptors only.
C. constricts the pupils.
D. causes glycogenolysis.
E. inhibits the mobilisation of free fatty acids.

24. Human placental lactogen

A. is a single-chain polypeptide.
B. reaches the same concentration in fetal and maternal blood at term.
C. may be secreted by the decidua.
D. is detectable only after the 25th week of pregnancy.
E. is an insulin antagonist.

25. Arginine vasopressin

A. reduces glomerular filtration rate.
B. controls water loss in the proximal renal tubule.
C. is synthesised by the posterior pituitary gland.
D. is released in response to a rise in plasma osmolality.
E. is released in response to a fall in circulating plasma volume.

26. In a healthy adult, serum calcium

A. constitutes 15% of total body calcium.
B. is not involved in the extrinsic system of blood coagulation.
C. concentration will be lowered by calcitonin.
D. concentration normally falls after the menopause.
E. is approximately 90% protein-bound.

27. Concerning the human ovary:

A. Aromatase catalyses the conversion of testosterone to 17β oestradiol.
B. Relaxin is synthesised in the corpus luteum.
C. Inhibin stimulates follicle-stimulating hormone release from the pituitary gland.
D. Progesterone decreases the sensitivity of myometrial cells to oxytocin.
E. Cholesterol is converted to androstenedione in granulosa cells.

28. Human chorionic gonadotrophin

A. is a glycoprotein.
B. secretion peaks at 20 weeks of gestation.
C. has intrinsic anti-thyroid activity.
D. is synthesised by the corpus luteum of pregnancy.
E. binds to luteinising hormone receptors.

29. Gonadotrophin-releasing hormone

A. is a dimeric glycoprotein.
B. is synthesised in the hypothalamus.
C. stimulates synthesis of follicle-stimulating hormone.
D. secretion is increased following castration.
E. pulsatile administration inhibits ovarian steroid production.

30. The following are RNA-containing viruses:

A. coxsackie.
B. influenza.

C. mumps.
D. herpes simplex.
E. cytomegalovirus.

31. Concerning viral infections:

A. Cytomegalovirus is of the herpes group.
B. Herpes simplex virus may remain dormant in epithelial cells of the lower genital tract.
C. Facial herpes simplex lesions are activated by sunlight.
D. Coxsackie B virus does not cross the placenta.
E. Hepatitis B virus may be sexually transmitted.

32. Exotoxins

A. are derived from Gram-negative bacteria.
B. have a specific action.
C. are more toxic than endotoxins.
D. are neutralised by their homologous antitoxin.
E. can be converted to toxoid.

33. Vesical schistosomiasis

A. is acquired by eating snails.
B. causes intermittent haematuria.
C. is diagnosed by finding schistosome eggs in the urine.
D. is endemic in South America.
E. is sexually transmitted.

34. Listeria monocytogenes

A. is a Gram-negative organism.
B. is sensitive to ampicillin.
C. may cause a transplacental infection.
D. is sexually transmitted.
E. can be cultured from a high vaginal swab.

35. Actinomyces israelii

A. is a fungus.
B. forms yellow granules in pus.
C. is a mouth commensal.
D. occurs in association with intrauterine contraceptive devices.
E. is resistant to penicillin.

36. Concerning syphilis:

A. The incubation period is usually between 1 and 7 days.
B. It has an infectious secondary stage.
C. The primary stage is characterised by gumma formation.
D. The Wassermann reaction becomes positive in the tertiary stage.
E. Haematogenous spread occurs early.

37. BCG vaccination of previously uninfected persons

A. produces local erythema within 24 hours.
B. results in regional lymph node enlargement.
C. produces a visible reaction within 3 days.
D. should be given intramuscularly.
E. is ineffective in the newborn.

38. The causative organism of

A. condylomata lata is *Neisseria gonorrhoeae*.
B. chancroid is *Haemophilus ducreyii*.
C. granuloma inguinalae is *Donovania granulomatis*.
D. primary chancre is *Treponema pertenue*.
E. yaws is *Gardnerella vaginalis*.

39. The following infectious diseases are arthropod-borne:

A. bubonic plague.
B. malaria.
C. legionnaire's disease.
D. yellow fever.
E. epidemic typhus fever.

40. The following drugs may cause enlargement of the fetal thyroid gland:

A. methyldopa.
B. thyroxine.
C. carbimazole.
D. propranolol.
E. propylthiouracil.

41. The following substances lower the blood glucose concentration:

A. adrenaline.
B. chlorpropamide.

C.   chlorothiazide.*
D.   metformin.
E.   thyroxine.

42. The following drugs stimulate myometrial contractility:

A.   vasopressin.
B.   nifedipine.
C.   hydralazine hydrochloride.
D.   salbutamol.
E.   indomethacin.

43. The following are beta-mimetic effects:

A.   constriction of bronchioles.
B.   increased heart rate.
C.   a decrease in the force of cardiac contraction.
D.   constriction of arterioles in the skin.
E.   increased glycogenolysis in skeletal muscle.

44. The following are features of ergometrine maleate:

A.   It is inactive when administered orally.
B.   The onset of action after intravenous injection occurs in
     approximately 5 minutes.
C.   Transient hypertension may occur after its administration.
D.   Parenteral administration may result in vomiting.
E.   Its use is contraindicated in patients with migraine.

45. Thiopentone sodium administered intravenously

A.   is a potent muscle relaxant.
B.   is predominantly excreted by the kidney.
C.   binds to protein.
D.   is fat soluble.
E.   crosses the placenta.

46. The following statements about anticoagulants are correct:

A.   Heparin inhibits the action of thrombin.
B.   The action of heparin is antagonised by vitamin K.
C.   Heparin increases antithrombin III activity.
D.   The effects of coumarin anticoagulants are decreased by metronidazole.
E.   Warfarin is greater than 80% protein-bound in plasma.

* This drug has now been discontinued in the UK.

47. The following stimulate peristalsis in the large bowel:

A. opiates.
B. liquid paraffin.
C. suxamethonium chloride.
D. neostigmine.
E. senna glycoside.

48. The following drugs and side effects are associated:

A. carbenoxolone : sodium retention.
B. chlorothiazide* : hypoglycaemia.
C. salbutamol : bronchospasm.
D. clonidine : rebound hypertension.
E. phenytoin : folate deficiency.

49. The following drugs and side effects are associated:

A. methyldopa : depression.
B. paracetamol : thromboembolism.
C. indomethacin : peptic ulcer.
D. prednisolone : osteoporosis.
E. ritodrine : hypoglycaemia.

50. A hundred women at high risk of ovarian carcinoma have a pelvic ultrasound scan. The findings after scan and surgery are shown in the table:

Pelvic scan	Ovarian cancer		Total (n)
	Present (n)	Absent (n)	
Abnormal	15	20	35
Normal	5	60	65
Total	20	80	100

A. The sensitivity of the scan is 25%.
B. The specificity of the scan is 75%.
C. The prevalence of ovarian carcinoma is 25%.
D. There are 15 true positive cases.
E. 75% of the patients with ovarian carcinoma had positive scans.

---

* This drug has now been discontinued in the UK.

September 1998 Paper 2

1.   Concerning folic acid:

A.   It is a water soluble vitamin.
B.   Conversion of dihydrofolate to tetrahydrofolate is inhibited by methotrexate.
C.   Red cell folate concentration can be reduced by phenytoin.
D.   Tetrahydrofolic acid is a carrier of one-carbon units.
E.   It is involved in the synthesis of purines.

2.   2,3-diphosphoglycerate

A.   is present at higher concentrations in maternal erythrocytes than fetal erythrocytes.
B.   binds more avidly to haemoglobin A than to haemoglobin F.
C.   increases the affinity of haemoglobin for oxygen.
D.   is a phospholipid.
E.   is synthesised by the pentose phosphate pathway.

3.   Haematopoiesis in the fetus

A.   results in nucleated erythrocytes early in development.
B.   occurs in the yolk sac in the first month.
C.   does not occur in the bone marrow until term.
D.   is predominantly hepatic during the 4th month.
E.   does not require folic acid.

4.   Iron

A.   is altered to the ferric state after absorption.
B.   is transported by apoferritin.
C.   is readily excreted by the kidney.
D.   retention in the body is enhanced by chelating agents.
E.   · requirement during normal pregnancy is approximately 1 mg per day.

5. Cholecalciferol (vitamin D)

A. promotes the absorption of calcium from the gut.
B. is 25-hydroxylated in the liver.
C. is synthesised in the skin.
D. is 1-hydroxylated in the kidney.
E. is most active in the 1,25-dihydroxyl form.

6. Excess

A. vitamin C causes haemorrhage.
B. vitamin D causes renal failure.
C. vitamin K causes thrombosis.
D. vitamin E causes azoospermia.
E. vitamin A causes headache.

7. Concerning carbon dioxide:

A. It is mainly carried in the blood as carbaminohaemoglobin.
B. 10–15% is carried in the blood in simple solution.
C. It diffuses across the placenta more readily than oxygen.
D. It is displaced more easily from fetal blood after oxygenation.
E. It is more soluble in body fluids than oxygen.

8. Chemicals are solubilised in the liver by

A. glucuronide formation.
B. transamination.
C. bile salt conjugation.
D. acetylation.
E. carboxylation.

9. Unconjugated bilirubin

A. is normally present in the plasma in lower concentration than conjugated bilirubin.
B. circulates in the plasma bound to albumin.
C. is not excreted in the urine.
D. does not cross the blood–brain barrier.
E. is bound to specific proteins in the liver cells.

10. Messenger ribonucleic acid (mRNA)

A. is a double-stranded polymer.
B. is transcribed from DNA in the nucleus.

C. is not present in reticulocytes.
D. contains thymine.
E. is not present in oocytes.

11. Glycogen

A. is a polymer of glucose residues.
B. is predominantly found in cytoplasm.
C. is mainly stored in the liver.
D. is cleaved by phosphorylase to glucose-1-phosphate.
E. breakdown is inhibited by adrenaline.

12. Hyperkalemia is a characteristic finding in

A. primary aldosteronism.
B. treatment with spironolactone.
C. hyperparathyroidism.
D. adrenocorticotrophic hormone-secreting tumours of the bronchus.
E. renal failure.

13. Glucose

A. is predominantly absorbed in the terminal ileum.
B. stimulates the secretion of glucagon.
C. can be synthesised from pyruvate.
D. is a disaccharide.
E. is the only metabolic substrate for cardiac muscle.

14. In an X-linked pedigree

A. none of the sons of an affected male will be affected.
B. half of the daughters of an affected male will not carry the gene.
C. half of the sons of carrier females will be affected.
D. females are never affected.
E. all of the daughters of a carrier female will themselves be carriers.

15. In the neonate, the appearance of the external genitalia may not correspond with the genotype in the presence of

A. adrenogenital syndrome.
B. testicular feminisation syndrome.
C. renal agenesis (Potter's syndrome).
D. trisomy 21.
E. severe hypospadias.

16. Chromosome analysis

A.   can be performed more quickly from chorionic villus samples than from amniotic fluid samples.
B.   is based entirely on assessment of chromosome size.
C.   is carried out at the metaphase stage of mitosis.
D.   of a classical hydatidiform mole is usually 46XX.
E.   of the fetus will be abnormal in about 80% of cases of exomphalos.

17. Concerning inheritable diseases:

A.   Huntingdon's chorea is transmitted by a dominant gene.
B.   Phenylketonuria is transmitted by a recessive gene.
C.   Haemophilia is an autosomal dominant condition.
D.   Von Willebrand's disease is a sex-linked condition.
E.   Cystic fibrosis is transmitted by an X-linked recessive gene.

18. Concerning immunoglobulins in pregnancy:

A.   Maternal IgM is responsible for rhesus isoimmunisation in the fetus.
B.   IgA concentration in cord blood is higher than that in maternal blood.
C.   IgE crosses the placenta readily.
D.   IgG crosses the placenta readily.
E.   Fetal IgM is dimeric.

19. Immunodeficiency states may be associated with

A.   viral infection of T lymphocytes.
B.   B cell lymphomata.
C.   glucocorticoid administration.
D.   haemolytic disease of the newborn.
E.   Hodgkin's lymphoma.

20. Early blood-borne dissemination is a characteristic feature of

A.   carcinoma of the endometrium.
B.   osteosarcoma.
C.   basal cell carcinoma.
D.   carcinoma of the cervix.
E.   choriocarcinoma.

21. In tissue pigmentation, the following are associated:

A.   kernicterus and conjugated bilirubin.

B.   Addison's disease and increased cutaneous melanin.
C.   melanosis coli and bile pigments.
D.   Wilson's disease and copper deposition in the cornea.
E.   corpus luteum and carotenoids.

22. The following cells may be phagocytic:

A.   neutrophils.
B.   Kupffer cells.
C.   monocytes.
D.   Hofbauer cells.
E.   plasma cells.

23. Metastatic calcification may be seen in the following conditions:

A.   old pulmonary tuberculosis.
B.   degenerating leiomyomata.
C.   multiple myeloma.
D.   hyperparathyroidism.
E.   sarcoidosis.

24. In healing by primary intention, the following events occur:

A.   formation of a fibrin-free haematoma.
B.   an acute inflammatory reaction.
C.   migration of epithelial cells within 6 hours.
D.   phagocytosis.
E.   invasion by capillary buds within three days.

25. Amyloid

A.   is predominantly intracellular.
B.   contains fibrils.
C.   is enzymatic.
D.   can be found in nerve tissue.
E.   deposits occur with chronic sepsis.

26. The following are premalignant conditions:

A.   diverticular disease of the large bowel.
B.   ulcerative colitis.
C.   pulmonary asbestosis.
D.   Paget's disease of the bone.
E.   condylomata lata of the vulva.

27. Tetany may occur as a complication of

A. osteoporosis.
B. hypercapnia.
C. respiratory acidosis.
D. peripheral neuropathy.
E. untreated hyperparathyroidism.

28. In tumours of bone,

A. primary malignancy is more common than secondary malignancy.
B. osteoma rarely present in skull bones.
C. osteosarcoma is associated with Paget's disease of bone.
D. lymph node metastases are unusual.
E. simple bone cysts have a strong tendency to recur.

29. Acquired diverticular disease of the colon

A. is present in at least 15% of Caucasians over the age of 50 years.
B. is due to a congenital abnormality of the bowel wall.
C. is associated with increased intraluminal pressure.
D. is associated with muscular thickening.
E. may result in intestinal obstruction.

30. Stored blood which is to be used for transfusion

A. is kept at $-4°C$.
B. must be used within 1 week.
C. is tested for complement content before transfusion.
D. may be used for platelet replacement.
E. contains an acid anticoagulant.

31. In uncomplicated homozygous beta thalassaemia there is

A. hypochromasia.
B. a reduction in haemoglobin A_2.
C. an increase in haemoglobin F.
D. megaloblastic erythropoiesis.
E. red cell sickling.

32. The following tissues are capable of cellular regeneration:

A. spinal cord.
B. liver.
C. epidermis.

D.   myocardium.
E.   bone marrow.

33. Concerning oxygenation of fetal blood:

A.   The fetal-maternal P_{CO_2} gradient facilitates maternal–fetal oxygen transfer.
B.   Fetal haemoglobin is less influenced by 2,3-diphosphoglyceric acid concentration than adult haemoglobin.
C.   The fetal blood oxygen dissociation curve lies to the right of the maternal curve.
D.   The uptake of oxygen decreases fetal red cell buffering capacity.
E.   Uptake of oxygen by fetal blood is associated with a shift of chloride into fetal red cells.

34. Concerning the fetal cardiovascular system:

A.   More than 80% of the cardiac output flows through the placenta.
B.   Oxygen saturation in the carotid and renal arteries is the same.
C.   Umbilical venous blood has a lower P_{O_2} than renal arterial blood.
D.   Blood from the inferior vena cava passes directly into the left ventricle.
E.   The pulmonary circulation has a high resistance.

35. The Leydig cells of the testis

A.   secrete seminal fluid.
B.   are stimulated by luteinising hormone.
C.   are active in intrauterine life.
D.   secrete fructose.
E.   produce androstenedione.

36. In the lungs of a healthy male adult at rest

A.   alveolar air contains 40% nitrogen.
B.   about 3 litres of air are in the alveoli at the end of a quiet expiration.
C.   about 150 ml of inspired air in each breath do not reach the alveoli.
D.   the oxygen tension of blood in the pulmonary vein is about 5.3 KPa (about 40 mmHg).
E.   inspiration is brought about by relaxation of the intercostal muscles.

37. In the nonpregnant woman, during the cardiac cycle

A.   atrial contraction occurs in the early stages of ventricular filling.
B.   adrenergic stimulation increases the heart rate.
C.   the first heart sound is caused by closure of the aortic valves.

D.   stroke volume at rest is 200 ml.
E.   the peak pressure in the pulmonary arterial system is less than one-tenth of that in the systemic circulation.

38. Intracellular concentration of free calcium

A.   is greater than that of extracellular free calcium.
B.   may be influenced by voltage-gated membrane channels.
C.   may be influenced by the activity of inositol triphosphate.
D.   binds to calmodulin.
E.   inactivates trophonin.

39. The blood concentrations of the following are lowered in pregnancy:

A.   bicarbonate.
B.   transferrin.
C.   sodium.
D.   albumin.
E.   fibrinogen.

40. Plasminogen is

A.   a globulin.
B.   activated by α_2-macroglobulin.
C.   inhibited by streptokinase.
D.   formed from plasmin.
E.   released from plasma cells.

41. Concerning a woman with blood group type A:

A.   She may have a genotype AB.
B.   Her father may be group O.
C.   All of her children will be group A or O.
D.   If her husband has blood group A, all of their children will have group A or O blood.
E.   She can be transfused safely with group AB blood.

42. Bile

A.   production is inhibited after vagal stimulation.
B.   is concentrated under the influence of secretin.
C.   has a pH of 5.5.
D.   is expelled from the gall bladder under the influence of cholecystokinin.
E.   normally contains high concentrations of free cholesterol.

43. During normal pregnancy, the maternal pituitary gland

A. becomes heavier.
B. doubles its production of follicle-stimulating hormone.
C. increases its secretion of alpha melanocyte-stimulating hormone.
D. decreases its rate of production of thyroid-stimulating hormone.
E. releases arginine vasopressin in response to an infusion of a hypertonic solution.

44. Thromboxane A$_2$

A. induces platelet aggregation.
B. has a half-life of about 30 minutes.
C. causes vasoconstriction.
D. is synthesised by the lipoxygenase pathway.
E. synthesis is inhibited by aspirin.

45. Angiotensin II

A. is a vasoconstrictor.
B. reduces aldosterone production.
C. is mainly found in the lungs.
D. is a decapeptide.
E. is produced when the extracellular fluid volume is reduced.

46. Bicarbonate

A. ions are reabsorbed from renal tubular fluid.
B. plasma concentration rises in respiratory acidosis.
C. plasma concentration falls in pregnancy.
D. in blood is predominantly carried by red cells.
E. is one of the unmeasured anions causing the 'anion gap'.

47. Total body water

A. forms a smaller proportion of body water in fat than thin persons.
B. can be measured by a deuterium oxide dilution technique.
C. normally comprises 45–65% of body weight.
D. Is a smaller proportion of body weight in men than in women.
E. Is predominantly intracellular.

48. Cardiac output in the adult

A. is greater from the left ventricle than from the right.
B. varies with physiological changes in the heart rate.

C. is reflexly reduced in a hot environment.
D. increases in the first trimester of pregnancy.
E. varies with stroke volume when the heart rate is constant.

49. During normal pregnancy the daily urinary excretion of

A. glucose is increased.
B. total amino acids is decreased.
C. total protein is decreased.
D. vitamin B_{12} is increased.
E. folate is decreased.

50. Physiological changes associated with pregnancy include

A. a rise in erythrocyte sedimentation rate.
B. a rise in total body haemoglobin.
C. a fall in plasma fibrinogen concentration.
D. an increase in the total number of leucocytes.
E. an increase in blood urea concentration within the first trimester.

March 1999
Paper 1

1. In the pituitary gland

A. the anterior lobe is smaller than the posterior lobe.
B. the posterior lobe is ectodermal in origin.
C. the acidophil cells produce oxytocin.
D. the basophil cells produce growth hormone.
E. the blood supply is derived from the internal carotid artery.

2. The following statements concerning the pelvic vessels are correct:

A. The inferior gluteal artery passes through the greater sciatic foramen.
B. The inferior vesical artery supplies the fundus of the bladder.
C. The middle rectal artery supplies the rectal mucosa.
D. The uterine venous plexus communicates with the rectal plexus.
E. The vesical venous plexus drains into the external iliac artery.

3. The obturator artery

A. branches from the posterior trunk of the internal iliac artery.
B. passes through the greater sciatic foramen.
C. is crossed by the ureter.
D. supplies the hip joint.
E. may be replaced by a branch of the superior epigastric artery.

4. The obturator nerve

A. arises from the sacral plexus.
B. descends through the psoas major muscle.
C. leaves the pelvis through the greater sciatic foramen.
D. mainly supplies the abductor muscles of the thigh.
E. innervates the obturator internus muscle.

5. The pelvic splanchnic nerves

A. supply the ascending colon.
B. contribute to the inferior hypogastric plexus.
C. are motor to the internal sphincter of the bladder.
D. contain afferent fibres for the ovary.
E. conduct pain from the body of the uterus.

6. The normal human preovulatory follicle

A. reaches a diameter of 40–60 mm before rupture.
B. requires luteinising hormone for development.
C. is lined by theca interna cells on its inner surface.
D. contains a zona-denuded oocyte.
E. contains fluid rich in progesterone.

7. In the pelvis, the ureter

A. is supplied by the uterine artery.
B. is crossed inferiorly by the uterine artery.
C. lies more than 5 cm lateral to the supravaginal cervix.
D. is derived from the urogenital sinus.
E. has sensory fibres passing in the pelvic splanchnic nerves.

8. In the femoral triangle, the femoral artery is

A. crossed by the superior circumflex iliac artery.
B. posterior to the femoral branch of the genitofemoral nerve.
C. medial to the long saphenous vein.
D. posterior to the femoral vein at the apex of the triangle.
E. medial to the femoral nerve.

9. The cervix

A. consists predominantly of smooth muscle.
B. is derived from mesoderm.
C. is covered by peritoneum on its anterior aspect.
D. is innervated by the pelvic splanchnic nerves.
E. is lined by keratinised epithelium.

10. The bladder

A. develops from the lower part of the urogenital sinus.
B. is supplied in part by the inferior epigastric artery.
C. drains lymph to the superficial inguinal nodes.

D.   is innervated by sympathetic fibres from segments T11 to L2.
E.   has a capacity of at least 1000 ml.

11. The following are derivatives of the mesonephros:

A.   appendix of the testis.
B.   efferent ductules of the testis.
C.   Gartner's duct cyst.
D.   gubernaculum testis.
E.   prostatic utricle.

12. The following are present in the developing umbilical cord:

A.   allantois.
B.   extra-embryonic mesoderm.
C.   intestinal loops.
D.   two umbilical arteries.
E.   yolk sac stalk.

13. During development of the female reproductive system

A.   primordial germ cells arise in the yolk sac.
B.   ovarian development is dependent upon oestrogen activity.
C.   the paramesonephric ducts give rise to the cervix.
D.   the greater vestibular glands arise from the urogenital sinus.
E.   differentiation of the external genitalia is dependent upon ovarian activity.

14. The fetal testes

A.   are morphologically distinguishable 4 weeks after conception.
B.   contain cells which have migrated from the wall of the yolk sac.
C.   are usually intra-abdominal 12 weeks after conception.
D.   are necessary for the persistence of the mesonephric (Wolffian) ducts.
E.   secrete androgens.

15. In a neonate at birth

A.   closure of the ductus arteriosus is due to increased arterial oxygen tension.
B.   the ductus arteriosus closes before the lungs are expanded.
C.   pressure in the inferior vena cava falls.
D.   the foramen ovale seals immediately.
E.   closure of the foramen ovale is due to increased carbon dioxide tension in venous blood.

16. Iodine

A. requirements are unchanged by pregnancy.
B. uptake by the thyroid gland is increased by thyroid-stimulating hormone.
C. is excreted by the kidney.
D. is bound to tyrosine in the thyroid gland.
E. may inhibit thyroxine synthesis.

17. The physiological action of oestradiol depends upon

A. metabolism to a more potent substance.
B. binding to an intracellular receptor.
C. alteration of gene expression.
D. active transport of the hormone into cells.
E. cyclic AMP production.

18. Testosterone in the human male

A. depresses pituitary secretion of luteinising hormone.
B. promotes growth of scalp hair.
C. promotes union of long-bone epiphyses.
D. is a more potent androgen than dihydrotestosterone.
E. is secreted maximally in the evening.

19. In congenital adrenal hyperplasia

A. the commonest cause is a deficiency of 21-hydroxylase.
B. the plasma cortisol concentration is increased.
C. there may be excessive secretion of 17α-hydroxyprogesterone.
D. sodium retention is characteristic.
E. blood catecholamine concentrations are increased.

20. The corpus luteum of pregnancy produces

A. relaxin.
B. progesterone.
C. 17α-hydroxyprogesterone.
D. human chorionic gonadotrophin.
E. oestradiol.

21. Concerning puberty in the female:

A. The development of secondary sexual characteristics is preceded by increased production of adrenal androgens.

B. Puberty is associated with the nocturnal release of luteinising hormone.
C. The ovaries are not sensitive to gonadotrophins before puberty.
D. Appearance of pubic hair usually precedes menarche.
E. Appearance of pubic hair precedes the onset of breast development.

22. Menopause

A. is due to failure of the endometrium to respond to oestrogens.
B. is associated with cessation of steroidogenesis within the ovary.
C. is associated with a fall in circulating luteinising hormone.
D. is preceded by a period of enhanced fertility.
E. results in atrophy of the epithelium of the distal urethra.

23. Products of human decidua include

A. α-fetoprotein.
B. prolactin.
C. human chorionic gonadotrophin.
D. human placental lactogen.
E. prostaglandin $F_{2\alpha}$.

24. Plasma levels of follicle-stimulating hormone are elevated in

A. adults with Klinefelter syndrome.
B. women taking oral contraceptive preparations.
C. postmenopausal women.
D. adults with Turner syndrome (45X0).
E. pregnancy.

25. Pituitary gonadotrophin

A. release is dependent upon hypothalamic function.
B. secretion increases during pregnancy.
C. blood levels are raised during lactational amenorrhoea.
D. release in the puerperium is enhanced by bromocriptine.
E. release is inhibited by oxytocin.

26. The release of catecholamines from the adrenal medulla increases

A. during sleep in healthy individuals.
B. when the nerves to the adrenal gland are stimulated.
C. when the blood sugar rises.
D. following myocardial infarction.
E. in the presence of a phaeochromocytoma.

27. Prolactin

A.   is secreted by the hypothalamus.
B.   plasma levels are raised in the first trimester of pregnancy.
C.   is identical to placental lactogen.
D.   controls milk ejection.
E.   release is inhibited by dopamine.

28. Human chorionic gonadotrophin

A.   has a half-life in blood of 2 hours.
B.   contains a beta chain indistinguishable from that of human luteinising hormone.
C.   is produced by the preimplantation blastocyst.
D.   is responsible for the maintenance of the corpus luteum in early pregnancy.
E.   may be produced in tissues other than trophoblast.

29. Growth hormone

A.   promotes protein synthesis.
B.   facilitates the hepatic synthesis of somatomedin C.
C.   promotes insulin-mediated uptake of glucose.
D.   increases circulating free fatty acids.
E.   stimulates epiphyseal fusion.

30. Antidiuretic hormone

A.   is normally synthesised in the hypothalamus.
B.   is secreted by the posterior pituitary gland.
C.   exerts its effect by reducing the glomerular filtration rate.
D.   is an oligopeptide.
E.   secretion is increased when plasma osmolality falls.

31. Calcitonin

A.   lowers the basal metabolic rate.
B.   concentration is increased in pregnancy.
C.   is released when the blood phosphate level rises.
D.   is produced in the thyroid gland.
E.   release is stimulated by high calcium ion levels.

32. The following hormones bind to receptors on the cell membrane:

A. corticosterone.
B. adrenaline.
C. luteinising hormone.
D. oestradiol.
E. gonadotrophin-releasing hormone.

33. *Schistosoma haematobium*

A. is a snail.
B. is prevalent in China.
C. infestation may affect the uterine cervix.
D. gives rise to chronic granulomatous lesions.
E. infestation predisposes to carcinoma.

34. Chlamydia organisms

A. are motile.
B. are intracellular.
C. infect squamous cells.
D. are found in birds.
E. cause trachoma.

35. *Candida albicans*

A. gives a positive reaction with Gram stain.
B. is an anaerobic organism.
C. is associated with diabetes mellitus.
D. is characterised by flagella.
E. is inhibited by oral tetracycline therapy.

36. Concerning Neisseria:

A. *N. meningitidis* can be a nasopharyngeal commensal.
B. *N. gonorrhoeae* will grow in anaerobic conditions.
C. *N. gonorrhoeae* culture is inhibited at low temperatures.
D. *N. gonorrhoeae* is identified within the cytoplasm of polymorphs.
E. *N. gonorrhoeae* infection can cause an arthropathy.

37. Mycobacteria are

A. acid-fast.
B. spore formers.
C. facultative anaerobes.
D. motile.
E. obligate intracellular parasites.

38. The following diseases and organisms are correctly paired:

A. chancroid : *Treponema pallidum*.
B. granuloma inguinale : *Donovania granulomatis*.
C. lymphogranuloma venereum : *Haemophilus ducreyii*.
D. gas gangrene : *Clostridium tetani*.
E. infectious mononucleosis : Epstein Barr virus.

39. The following diseases are correctly paired with their vectors:

A. toxoplasmosis : domestic cat.
B. leishmaniasis : house fly.
C. yellow fever : mosquito.
D. epidemic typhus : body louse.
E. leptospirosis : brown rat.

40. An oncogenic DNA virus

A. contains reverse transcriptase.
B. induces cellular transformation.
C. is implicated in the pathogenesis of Burkitt's lymphoma.
D. integrates into the host genome.
E. induces squamous papillomas of the skin in humans.

41. Cyproterone acetate

A. is an oestrogen.
B. is used for the treatment of amenorrhoea.
C. binds to androgen receptors.
D. increases libido.
E. inhibits spermatogenesis.

42. Propranolol

A. is a selective beta-adrenergic blocking agent.
B. is not secreted in breast milk.
C. given in pregnancy slows the maternal heart rate.
D. causes bad dreams.
E. antagonises the tocolytic effect of salbutamol.

43. Aspirin

A. inhibits cyclooxygenase.
B. is the treatment of choice in childhood fever.
C. is contraindicated in gout.

D.   should be avoided by women on anticoagulant therapy.
E.   has little anti-platelet activity when given in low dosage.

44.   Parenteral administration of atropine in therapeutic doses to a normal person causes

A.   impaired visual accommodation.
B.   diarrhoea.
C.   constriction of the bronchi.
D.   an increase in heart rate.
E.   a reduction in bronchial secretions.

45.   The following statements about morphine are true:

A.   All of its pharmacological actions are reversed by naloxone.
B.   It is transferred into breast milk.
C.   It does not cross the placenta in significant quantities.
D.   Its analgesic effects last about 1 hour.
E.   It causes pupillary dilatation.

46.   Lignocaine used as a local anaesthetic

A.   causes tachycardia if given as a systemic injection.
B.   has a longer lasting action than bupivicaine.
C.   is used in combination with adrenaline for ring block.
D.   causes vasoconstriction.
E.   is a weak base.

47.   The following statements about drug interactions are correct:

A.   Antacids decrease intestinal absorption of tetracyclines.
B.   The effects of warfarin are potentiated by combined oral contraceptives.
C.   The action of heparin is opposed by vitamin K.
D.   Alcohol metabolism is impaired by metronidazole.
E.   The effects of bromocriptine are potentiated by chlorpromazine.

48.   The following anti-hypertensive agents are correctly paired with their mode of action:

A.   captopril : angiotensin-converting enzyme inhibition.
B.   phentolamine : alpha-adrenoceptor blockade.
C.   methyldopa : ganglion blockade.
D.   hydralazine hydrochloride : angiotensin II inhibition.
E.   sodium nitroprusside : vasodilatation.

49. In a sample of 1000 children, the birth weight was normally distributed with a mean of 3.5 kg and a standard deviation of 700 g.

A. 15 infants would be below the 5th centile for weight.
B. The standard error of the birth weight would be about 22 g.
C. The 95th centile for birth weight would be 4.2 kg.
D. No baby would weigh less than 1.4 kg.
E. The median birth weight would be about 3.5 kg.

50. In a clinical trial, randomised allocation of patients to treatment groups

A. eliminates investigator bias.
B. reduces the placebo effect.
C. usually controls for known confounding variables.
D. usually controls for unknown confounding variables.
E. is best achieved by alternate allocation of subjects.

March 1999 Paper 2

1. **The conversion of glucose to lactic acid**

A. occurs in a single enzymatic reaction.
B. is the only pathway for the synthesis of ATP in the red blood cell.
C. is a reversible process in skeletal muscle.
D. is inhibited by high cellular concentrations of ATP.
E. occurs in skeletal muscle when the availability of oxygen is limited.

2. **Ketone bodies**

A. can be utilised by the fetal brain.
B. include acetoacetate.
C. are water soluble.
D. are synthesised in skeletal muscle.
E. can be utilised during starvation.

3. **Noradrenaline**

A. is a derivative of arginine.
B. is a precursor of adrenaline.
C. acts predominantly on alpha receptors.
D. is catabolised to vanillylmandelic acid.
E. Is metabolised by catechol-O-methyl transferase.

4. **ABO antigens are**

A. glycoproteins.
B. found only on erythrocytes.
C. major histocompatibility antigens.
D. not immunogenic during pregnancy.
E. located on membranes.

5. Nitrogen balance is

A. positive during pregnancy.
B. positive during prolonged immobilisation.
C. negative during protein starvation.
D. negative in the untreated diabetic.
E. positive during recovery from debilitating illness.

6. In the fetal lung

A. bronchial cartilage formation commences at 18–24 weeks of gestation.
B. type II alveolar cells first appear at 16–20 weeks gestation.
C. sphingomyelin is the most common phospholipid present at term.
D. phospholipid release is increased by endogenous adrenaline.
E. phospholipid production is decreased by exogenous corticosteroids.

7. Concerning acidosis:

A. The ratio of bicarbonate ions to carbonic acid in extracellular fluid is decreased.
B. In respiratory acidosis there is reduced renal hydrogen ion secretion.
C. In respiratory acidosis there is an increased concentration of carbon dioxide in the blood.
D. Loss of bicarbonate in diarrhoea causes a metabolic acidosis.
E. In compensating metabolic acidosis, Pco_2 is increased.

8. Fetal haemoglobin

A. contains four polypeptide chains.
B. does not contain iron.
C. has no alpha chains.
D. is more resistant to alkaline denaturation than is adult haemoglobin.
E. has the same structure as adult myoglobin.

9. The intestinal absorption of calcium is

A. decreased in renal failure.
B. decreased by the ingestion of large amounts of some cereals.
C. increased by the oral intake of phosphate.
D. increased by 1,25-dihydroxycholecalciferol.
E. decreased in the presence of steatorrhoea.

10. The following are amino acids found in human proteins

A. serine.
B. methionine.
C. thyramine.

D.   histamine.
E.   arginine.

11. Iron ions

A.   diffuse passively into erythropoietic cells.
B.   bind to transferrin.
C.   are taken up by hepatocytes.
D.   are necessary for cytochrome synthesis.
E.   are absorbed predominantly by the ileum.

12. Folic acid

A.   requires gastric intrinsic factor for its absorption.
B.   daily requirement is about 40 mg.
C.   is found in higher concentration in fetal blood than in maternal blood.
D.   deficiency leads to microcytic anaemia.
E.   is fat soluble.

13. Concerning immunoglobulins in pregnancy:

A.   The concentration of IgG is ten times greater in the maternal circulation than it is in the fetal circulation at term.
B.   The concentration of IgA in cord blood is higher than that in maternal blood.
C.   IgE crosses the placenta readily.
D.   The four classes of IgG cross the placenta readily.
E.   Fetal IgM is dimeric.

14. The conjugation of bilirubin

A.   takes place in hepatocytes.
B.   is catalysed by UDP glucuronyl transferase.
C.   is inhibited by phenobarbitone.
D.   renders it water soluble.
E.   is impaired in acute biliary obstruction.

15. In radiotherapy

A.   1 Gray is equivalent to 1 joule per kilogram.
B.   the skin usually receives a greater dose of radiation than the underlying tissues.
C.   the major effect of radiation energy is to damage the cytoplasm of the cell.

D.   cells in tissues which are hypoxic are more vulnerable to radiation.

E.   radiation-induced changes in tissues may take 6 weeks to develop.

16. In uncomplicated homozygous beta thalassaemia there is

A.   hypochromasia.
B.   a reduction in haemoglobin A_2.
C.   an increase in haemoglobin F.
D.   megaloblastic erythropoiesis.
E.   red cell sickling.

17. Concerning the genetic control of protein synthesis:

A.   Mature mRNA contains introns.
B.   A codon has 3-base sequences.
C.   Each amino acid has a single codon.
D.   Transfer RNA (tRNA) has anticodon recognition sites.
E.   Each tRNA carries a specific amino acid.

18. Concerning chromosomal errors:

A.   Structural variations may not have a phenotypic consequence.
B.   Trisomy indicates the presence of three haploid components within a cell.
C.   Nondisjunction during mitosis can contribute to mosaicism.
D.   A trisomic parent can produce normal gametes.
E.   Triploidy is rarely detected in neonates at term.

19. The following conditions are hereditary:

A.   polyposis coli.
B.   retinoblastorna.
C.   xeroderma pigmentosa.
D.   Burkitt's lymphoma.
E.   osteosarcoma.

20. Immunoglobulin M

A.   fixes complement by the alternative pathway.
B.   crosses the placenta readily.
C.   fixes to mast cells.
D.   is produced by plasma cells.
E.   is smaller than immunoglobulin E.

21. **Lymphocytes in health**

A. form about 2% of the white cell count.
B. play an essential role in cell mediated immunity.
C. can change into plasma cells.
D. have proportionately more nuclear material than cytoplasm.
E. have a life span of about 30 days.

22. **In anaphylactic shock in humans**

A. IgE is a mediator.
B. there is degranulation of mast cells.
C. complement is required.
D. histamine release occurs.
E. the principle response is in the gastrointestinal tract.

23. **Concerning the adrenal gland:**

A. The cortex is derived from neural crest cells.
B. The zona fasciculata secretes aldosterone.
C. Cortical adenomas may cause Cushing syndrome.
D. Neuroblastomas arise in the medulla.
E. Addison's disease may result from autoimmune destruction of the cortex.

24. **The following are autosomal recessive diseases:**

A. neurofibromatosis.
B. cystic fibrosis.
C. phenylketonuria.
D. polyposis coli.
E. sickle cell anaemia.

25. **The following are examples of type-III hypersensitivity (immune-complex) diseases:**

A. autoimmune haemolytic anaemia.
B. systemic lupus erythematosus.
C. glomerulonephritis.
D. tuberculosis.
E. sarcoidosis.

26. **The following tumours produce characteristic blood markers:**

A.   clear cell carcinoma.
B.   choriocarcinoma.
C.   osteogenic sarcoma.
D.   yolk sac tumour.
E.   transitional cell tumour.

27. **Uterine fibroids**

A.   are defined histologically as fibromyxomas.
B.   arise from endometrial stroma.
C.   may be associated with polycythaemia.
D.   predispose to endometrial hyperplasia.
E.   are liable to sarcomatous change in about 5% of cases.

28. **The following pairs indicate correct pathological association:**

A.   Epstein-Barr virus : Burkitt's lymphoma.
B.   Peutz-Jeghers syndrome : intestinal carcinoma.
C.   wood dust : pleural mesothelioma.
D.   progestagens : endometrial carcinoma.
E.   aniline dyes : bladder carcinoma.

29. **Obstruction of the lower end of the common bile duct is suggested by**

A.   an elevated serum conjugated bilirubin concentration.
B.   a reduced serum alkaline phosphatase concentration.
C.   the presence of urobilinogen in the urine.
D.   increased conjugated bilirubin in the urine.
E.   a reduced serum cholesterol concentration.

30. **Growth of the following tumours is hormone dependent:**

A.   squamous cell carcinoma of the cervix.
B.   breast adenocarcinoma.
C.   uterine leiomyoma.
D.   prostatic adenocarcinoma.
E.   testicular carcinoma.

31. **Osteomalacia is characterised by**

A.   mineralisation of the periosteum.
B.   deposition of uncalcified bone matrix.
C.   normal osteoblastic activity.

D. increased capillary fragility.
E. normal calcification of bone.

32. The following cause platelet aggregation

A. ADP (adenosine diphosphate).
B. prostacyclin.
C. serotonin.
D. antithrombin III.
E. thromboxane A_2.

33. Oxygen

A. binds to trivalent iron in the haem molecule.
B. is carried as four molecules per molecule of haemoglobin.
C. - haemoglobin dissociation is linear.
D. uptake reduces red cell buffering capacity.
E. is released from haemoglobin when the concentration of 2,3-diphosphoglyceric acid is decreased.

34. Displacement of oxyhaemoglobin dissociation to the right

A. means a greater avidity of haemoglobin for oxygen.
B. occurs immediately on ascent to high altitude.
C. occurs with a rise in temperature.
D. occurs with a fall in pH.
E. occurs with a fall in Pco_2.

35. Plasma osmolarity in the human

A. is normally about 290 milliosmoles per kg in the nonpregnant state.
B. increases during the first trimester of pregnancy.
C. is closely controlled by plasma protein concentration.
D. is regulated by arginine vasopressin.
E. regulates the sensation of thirst.

36. Gastrointestinal absorption of

A. dietary glucose depends upon intact pancreatic function.
B. vitamin B_{12} requires gastric acid.
C. fats is accomplished by the transport of chylomicrons from the intestinal lumen.
D. iron may be reduced by vitamin C administration.
E. unhydrolised polysaccharides does not occur.

37. In the healthy adult kidney

A. glucose resorption predominantly occurs in the loop of Henle.
B. water is reabsorbed in the proximal tubule by active transport.
C. the glomerular filtration rate is 25 ml per minute.
D. resorption of sodium is increased by aldosterone.
E. urinary pH can vary between 4.5 and 8.5.

38. Plasma proteins

A. which combine with drugs enhance their pharmacological activity.
B. play no role in the plasma buffering system.
C. combine with lipids to facilitate transport.
D. are restored within 24 hours after haemorrhage.
E. are normally present in a concentration of about 7g/l.

39. Surfactant

A. is formed mainly in the placenta.
B. levels in amniotic fluid diminish after 33 weeks of gestation.
C. formation can be inferred from the lecithin–sphingomyelin ratio in amniotic fluid.
D. contains palmitic acid.
E. decreases the surface tension in pulmonary alveoli.

40. The normal human erythrocyte

A. has an average volume of 70 fl.
B. is spherical.
C. has a diameter of 10 micrometres.
D. has a survival time of about 120 days.
E. has a haemoglobin content of less than 40%.

41. Concerning nitrogen metabolism:

A. Ingestion of complex proteins is essential for the maintenance of nitrogen balance.
B. There are eight essential amino acids.
C. The minimum daily requirement of each essential amino acid is 0.3–1.0 g.
D. Amino acid nitrogen is largely excreted as urea.
E. A protein poor, but energy sufficient diet will cause a decreased excretion of creatinine.

42. A woman has the following blood gas profile: pH = 7.6, P_{CO_2} = 2.7 KPa (20 mmHg), standard bicarbonate = 27 mmol/l.

A. These figures are compatible with normal pregnancy.
B. She could be hyperventilating.
C. She could have diabetic ketoacidosis.
D. The alveolar P_{CO_2} would be 6.3 KPa (47 mmHg).
E. The plasma hydrogen ion concentration would be 0.000076 mmol/l.

43. Nerve impulses

A. can only travel in one direction along an axon.
B. require energy.
C. are conducted at approximately the speed of light.
D. are conducted at the same speed in small and large axons.
E. are not delayed at the synapse before transmission.

44. Intracellular fluid differs from extracellular fluid in that

A. it forms the major proportion of total body water.
B. its volume can be measured easily.
C. it has a higher concentration of potassium than of sodium.
D. its volume is regulated primarily by the kidneys.
E. it has a higher phosphate concentration.

45. In the conducting system of the normal heart

A. the cardiac impulse originates in the atrioventricular (AV) node.
B. the AV node is situated in the wall of the coronary sinus.
C. Purkinje fibres are modified muscle cells.
D. the AV bundle lies in the interventricular septum.
E. the AV bundle divides to supply each ventricle.

46. Hypotension causes

A. diminished urine production.
B. inhibition of renin secretion.
C. stimulation of aldosterone secretion.
D. stimulation of angiotensin II production.
E. increased excretion of sodium.

47. During the fifth month of pregnancy, fetal red cell production normally occurs in the

A. lymph glands.
B. Kupffer cells of the liver.

C. bone marrow.
D. spleen.
E. placenta.

48. Myometrial activity in pregnancy is

A. increased by oestrogens.
B. increased by progesterone.
C. stimulated by vasopressin.
D. inhibited by ergot alkaloids.
E. inhibited by salbutamol.

49. By the 12th week of pregnancy, the following alterations have occurred

A. an increase in urea excretion.
B. a decrease in serum creatinine concentration.
C. diminished excretion of water soluble vitamins.
D. a doubling of 24-hour urinary volume.
E. an increase of serum urate concentration.

50. In pregnancy,

A. red cell mass increases.
B. serum iron binding capacity is decreased.
C. plasma folate levels are reduced.
D. respiration rate is increased.
E. lung tidal volume is increased.

September 1999 Paper 1

1. **Concerning oogenesis:**

A. The primary oogonia undergo mitotic divisions prior to meiosis.
B. The primary oocytes enter meiosis at puberty.
C. At birth, primary oocytes have completed the first meiotic division.
D. DNA synthesis does not take place as part of the second meiotic division.
E. Secondary oocytes complete the second meiotic division at ovulation.

2. **In the vulva,**

A. sebaceous glands are not present in the labia minora.
B. apocrine glands are present in the labia majora.
C. both surfaces of the hymen are covered by keratinised epithelium.
D. the Bartholin's glands are mucus-secreting.
E. the clitoris is covered by columnar epithelium.

3. **The anal canal**

A. has an upper part which is innervated by the inferior hypogastric plexus.
B. has a lower part which is supplied by the superior rectal artery.
C. drains lymph to the superficial inguinal nodes from its upper part.
D. has its internal sphincter innervated by the inferior rectal nerve.
E. has a superficial part of its external sphincter attached to the coccyx.

4. **The adult pituitary gland**

A. contains the paraventricular nuclei.
B. is related to the sphenoid bone.
C. lies inferiorly to the optic chiasma.
D. contains a pars tuberalis inferiorly.
E. is entirely ectodermal in origin.

5. The right ovarian artery

A. arises from the abdominal aorta above the renal artery.
B. passes posterior to the third (horizontal) part of the duodenum.
C. passes posterior to the genitofemoral nerve.
D. supplies the right ureter.
E. anastomoses with the right uterine artery.

6. The obturator nerve

A. is derived in part from the second lumbar nerve.
B. supplies both hip and knee joints.
C. runs superficial to the common iliac vessels.
D. leaves the pelvis through the greater sciatic foramen.
E. supplies the abductor muscles of the thigh.

7. Regarding the innervation of the genital tract

A. pre-ganglionic sympathetic nerves to the cervix arise from S2, S3 and S4.
B. pre-ganglionic sympathetic nerves to the body of the uterus arise from T12 and L1.
C. sensory nerves from the body of the uterus enter T11 and T12.
D. sensory nerves from the cervix enter S2, S3 and S4.
E. sensory nerves from the vagina enter L5 and S1.

8. The extradural (epidural) space

A. contains the internal vertebral plexus.
B. lies between the pia mater and dura mater.
C. contains no cerebrospinal fluid.
D. ends at the level of the second lumbar vertebra.
E. does not extend laterally through the intervertebral foramina.

9. The mature ovary

A. is attached to the anterior aspect of the broad ligament by the mesovarium.
B. is covered by a thick capsule.
C. has a surface layer of germinal epithelium.
D. on the right side drains venous blood to the renal vein.
E. has lymphatics which pass to external iliac nodes.

10. The vagina

A. has an anterior wall longer than the posterior wall.
B. contains mucus-secreting glands in its epithelium.
C. is related in its lower third to the bladder base.
D. during reproductive life has an acid pH.
E. is derived from the mesonephric duct.

11. The right ureter

A. is approximately 50 cm in length.
B. is partly covered by the duodenum.
C. crosses the genitofemoral nerve.
D. enters the bladder anteromedially.
E. receives part of its blood supply from the uterine artery.

12. Concerning the inguinal canal:

A. It transmits the ilioinguinal nerve.
B. The deep inguinal ring lies below the mid point of the inguinal ligament.
C. The superficial inguinal ring overlies the pubic tubercle.
D. Medially, the anterior wall is made up of the external oblique aponeurosis.
E. Laterally, the posterior wall is formed by the conjoint tendon.

13. After birth,

A. the allantois forms the median umbilical ligament.
B. the umbilical vein forms the medial umbilical ligament.
C. the umbilical artery forms the superior vesical artery.
D. the ductus venosus forms the ligamentum teres.
E. the ductus arteriosus forms the arch of the aorta.

14. The normal neonate delivered at term has

A. a head circumference of between 40 cm and 50 cm.
B. a liver palpable on abdominal examination.
C. a blood glucose concentration above 1.66 mmol/l (30 g/dl).
D. brown adipose tissue.
E. no adult haemoglobin.

15. In spermatogenesis,

A.   primary spermatocytes undergo reduction division.
B.   each primary spermatocyte ultimately gives rise to four spermatids.
C.   the whole process of spermatogenesis in man takes 6–7 days.
D.   grossly abnormal spermatozoa may be found in fertile semen.
E.   spermatids are haploid.

16. Corticotrophin-releasing hormone

A.   is a polypeptide.
B.   is released from the median eminence of the hypothalamus.
C.   acts on the basophil cells of the anterior pituitary.
D.   release has a circadian variation.
E.   release is increased by painful stimuli.

17. Inhibin

A.   is structurally identical to relaxin.
B.   is released in pulses.
C.   is a steroid.
D.   is produced by the ovarian follicle.
E.   inhibits the release of follicle-stimulating hormone.

18. In the human male, dihydrotestosterone

A.   is a precursor of testosterone.
B.   has one-tenth of the potency of testosterone.
C.   is responsible for involution of the Müllerian system.
D.   is responsible for the development of the male external genitalia.
E.   binds to an intracellular receptor.

19. In human lactation

A.   oestrogens promote development of the breast lobules.
B.   oestrogens promote the milk-producing effect of prolactin on the breast.
C.   human placental lactogen is essential for milk synthesis.
D.   prolactin stimulates gonadotrophin release.
E.   oxytocin causes milk ejection.

20. Aldosterone

A.   secretion is increased by a low potassium intake.
B.   production is reduced in normal pregnancy.

C.   secretion is entirely regulated by the rennin–angiotensin system.
D.   is the principle mineralocorticoid secreted by the adrenal gland.
E.   in the kidney, acts on the distal convoluted tubule.

21. In the renin-angiotensin system

A.   decreased renal blood flow causes increased renin production.
B.   renin is secreted by the juxta-glomerular cells of the kidney.
C.   renin causes production of angiotensin I.
D.   angiotensin I is a decapeptide.
E.   angiotensin II suppresses aldosterone secretion.

22. Concerning insulin:

A.   The half-life of endogenous insulin in the circulation is 30 minutes.
B.   The kidney is a major site of insulin degradation.
C.   It facilitates glucose uptake by the brain.
D.   Fasting concentrations are lower in pregnant women at term than
     they are in nonpregnant women.
E.   It is formed when C-peptide is separated from proinsulin.

23. During normal pregnancy

A.   plasma thyroid-binding globulin concentration increases.
B.   plasma total thyroxine concentration falls.
C.   plasma TSH concentration increases.
D.   triiodothyronine readily crosses the placenta to the fetus.
E.   fetal thyroid function is largely dependent upon the function of the
     maternal thyroid.

24. Concerning testicular hormones:

A.   Testosterone reduces plasma luteinising hormone concentrations.
B.   Inhibin stimulates luteinising hormone production.
C.   Oestrogens are formed in the testis.
D.   Testosterone is converted to dihydrotestosterone by 5α-reductase.
E.   Testosterone in plasma is predominantly bound to albumin.

25. Deficient adrenocortical function causes an increase in

A.   blood pressure.
B.   blood glucose.
C.   skin pigmentation.
D.   serum sodium.
E.   plasma lipids.

26. Progesterone

A.   is a C-21 steroid.
B.   is synthesised by the ovary before ovulation.
C.   increases ventilation.
D.   raises basal body temperature.
E.   binds to corticotrophin-binding globulin.

27.   Luteinising hormone

A.   is a glycoprotein.
B.   has a molecular weight of approximately 4000 Daltons.
C.   stimulates androgen production by the ovary.
D.   concentrations in the circulation are high in girls before puberty.
E.   concentrations in the circulation are raised in untreated adults with Turner syndrome.

28.   Serum concentrations of follicle-stimulating hormone are

A.   increased in Kleinfelter syndrome.
B.   decreased in primary hypogonadism.
C.   decreased following the menopause.
D.   increased with oestrogen therapy.
E.   increased following male castration.

29.   Human chorionic gonadotrophin

A.   is a steroid hormone.
B.   is partly metabolised in the kidneys.
C.   has an alpha subunit which is antigenically similar to the beta subunit of luteinising hormone.
D.   reaches peak concentrations at the 17th week of pregnancy.
E.   is secreted in trophoblastic disease.

30.   The secretion of growth hormone

A.   occurs in the hypothalamus.
B.   decreases during sleep.
C.   is decreased during stress.
D.   is decreased with hypoglycaemia.
E.   opposes the action of insulin.

31.   In the human, oxytocin

A.   promotes milk synthesis in the breast.

B. release is inhibited by alcohol.
C. action on the uterus is enhanced by oestrogens.
D. release is inhibited by dopamine.
E. in excess causes dehydration.

32. Calcitonin

A. increases the basal metabolic rate.
B. increases the blood calcium level.
C. is a steroid hormone.
D. is produced in the parathyroid glands.
E. release is stimulated by low calcium ion levels.

33. The pineal gland

A. lies anteriorly to the third ventricle.
B. is innervated by the parasympathetic nervous system.
C. produces melatonin.
D. increases in size at puberty.
E. activity is related to day length.

34. The following are RNA-containing viruses:

A. coxsackie.
B. influenza.
C. mumps.
D. herpes simplex.
E. cytomegalovirus.

35. Concerning viral infections:

A. Cytomegalovirus is of the herpes group.
B. Herpes simplex virus may remain dormant in epithelial cells of the lower genital tract.
C. Facial herpes simplex lesions are activated by sunlight.
D. Coxsackie B virus does not cross the placenta.
E. Hepatitis B virus may be sexually transmitted.

36. Bacteroides organisms

A. are motile.
B. do not produce spores.
C. grow in aerobic culture.
D. are synergistic coliforms.
E. are characteristically resistant to penicillin.

37. *Staphylococcus aureus*

A. produces coagulase.
B. is motile.
C. produces spores.
D. produces pigmented colonies.
E. produces toxins.

38. Mycoplasmas

A. are the smallest known free-living organisms.
B. have a typical bacterial cell wall.
C. are sensitive to penicillin.
D. are resistant to tetracycline.
E. can only be grown in tissue culture cells.

39. *Actinomyces israelii*

A. is a fungus.
B. forms yellow granules in pus.
C. is a mouth commensal.
D. occurs in association with intrauterine contraceptive devices.
E. is resistant to penicillin.

40. Concerning syphilis:

A. The incubation period is usually between 1 and 7 days.
B. It has an infectious secondary stage.
C. The primary stage is characterised by gumma formation.
D. The regain test becomes positive in the tertiary stage.
E. Haematogenous spread occurs early.

41. The discharge associated with bacterial vaginosis

A. contains clue 'cells'.
B. contains large numbers of polymorphs.
C. has a pH above 4.5.
D. is frothy.
E. has an odour.

42. The following factors enhance the transplacental passage of drugs:

A. lipid solubility.
B. a high degree of ionic dissociation.

C. high molecular weight.
D. protein binding.
E. uterine contractions.

43. The following drugs are potassium-sparing diuretics:

A. amiloride hydrochloride.
B. triamterene.
C. spironolactone.
D. chlorothiazide.*
E. frusemide.**

44. Metronidazole

A. is a folic acid antagonist.
B. is ineffective when given per rectum.
C. should not be administered intravenously.
D. is effective against *Entamoeba histolytica*.
E. interferes with ethanol metabolism.

45. The following agents inhibit uterine activity:

A. magnesium sulphate.
B. ritodrine hydrochloride.
C. oxprenolol hydrochloride.
D. fenoterol hydrobromide.
E. indomethacin.

46. The following drugs diminish detrusor contractions:

A. atropine.
B. carbachol.
C. propantheline.
D. nifedipine.
E. distigmine.

47. The following drugs are beta-sympathomimetic agonists:

A. adrenaline.
B. noradrenaline.
C. phenylephrine.
D. ritodrine hydrochloride.
E. oxprenolol hydrochloride.

---

* This drug has now been discontinued in the UK.
** Registered international non-proprietary is furosemide; BNF 48, September 2004.

48. The following drug combinations have been shown to interact to produce the stated effects:

A. ampicillin enhances the anticoagulant action of warfarin.
B. aciclovir diminishes the effect of oral contraceptives.
C. cimetidine inhibits the metabolism of phenytoin.
D. aspirin diminishes the action of ritodrine.
E. tamoxifen increases the anticoagulant effect of warfarin.

49. The following substances lower the blood glucose concentration:

A. adrenaline.
B. chlorpropamide.
C. chlorothiazide.*
D. metformin.
E. thyroxine.

50. Concerning the analysis of clinical trials:

A. The 95% confidence interval indicates the range within which 19 out of 20 values will lie.
B. The P value illustrates how often the result would be expected to occur by chance.
C. The conventional level of statistical significance is set at $P < 0.005$.
D. In a randomised trial, there must be equal numbers of recruits in each arm of the study.
E. A relative risk reduction of 60% is significant irrespective of the value of P.

* This drug has now been discontinued in the UK.

September 1999 Paper 2

1. Epidermal growth factor

A. is mitogenic.
B. synthesis is stimulated by oestradiol.
C. is a steroid molecule.
D. is found in endometrium.
E. binds to a receptor on the nuclear membrane.

2. Intracellular fluid differs from extracellular fluid in that

A. it forms the larger proportion of total body water.
B. its volume can be more readily measured.
C. it has a higher concentration of potassium.
D. its volume is more directly regulated by the kidneys.
E. it has a lower concentration of sodium.

3. Injected histamine produces

A. a fall in blood pressure.
B. decreased gastric secretion of hydrochloric acid.
C. bronchodilation.
D. bradycardia.
E. peripheral vasoconstriction.

4. The following are disaccharides:

A. glucose.
B. maltose.
C. sucrose.
D. fructose.
E. lactose.

5. The following are actively transported across the placenta from the maternal to the fetal circulation:

A. histidine.
B. alcohol.
C. ascorbic acid.
D. iron.
E. intrinsic factor.

6. Urea

A. is formed mainly in the kidney.
B. contains two amine (NH2) groups.
C. is formed by transamination from ketoglutarate.
D. is an end product of nitrogen metabolism in the fetus.
E. excretion is unrelated to protein intake.

7. Concerning amniotic fluid:

A. It has a protein concentration similar to that of maternal plasma.
B. It is mainly a filtrate of maternal plasma during the second half of pregnancy.
C. The highest bilirubin concentrations occur during the last trimester.
D. There is an increase in the α-fetoprotein concentration throughout pregnancy.
E. It contains cells of maternal origin.

8. Concerning the absorption of fats:

A. There is a major degree of lipase activity in the stomach.
B. Pancreatic lipase is the most important enzyme for fat digestion.
C. Bile salts contribute to the formation of micelles.
D. Micelles have a hydrophobic coat.
E. Chylomicrons have a core of triglycerides.

9. Ketone bodies

A. are synthesised in the brain.
B. include aceto-acetate.
C. are water soluble.
D. are synthesised in skeletal muscle.
E. can be utilised during starvation.

10. Serum alkaline phosphatase activity characteristically is raised in

A. senile osteoporosis.
B. intrahepatic cholestasis.
C. extensive Paget's disease of bone.
D. prostatic carcinoma.
E. pregnancy.

11. Vitamin A

A. can be synthesised in the skin.
B. is derived from β-carotene.
C. is toxic to tissues in high doses.
D. is a teratogen.
E. is required for rhodopsin synthesis.

12. The normal metabolic response to an operation includes

A. increased diuresis during the first 24 hours.
B. renal retention of sodium.
C. a rise in the plasma sodium level.
D. increased renal excretion of nitrogen.
E. increased renal excretion of potassium.

13. Folic acid

A. deficiency causes a megaloblastic bone marrow.
B. is hydroxycobalamin.
C. is present in green vegetables.
D. is predominantly absorbed from the large intestine.
E. is destroyed by boiling water.

14. In iodine metabolism

A. a daily intake of 100 mg of iodine is required to prevent goitre.
B. inorganic iodine is actively trapped by the thyroid gland.
C. iodine trapping is stimulated by thyroid-stimulating hormone.
D. iodine trapping is stimulated by perchlorate ion.
E. clearance of iodine by the thyroid is decreased during pregnancy.

15. The following are essential amino acids:

A. valine.
B. thiamine.

C.   cystamine.
D.   glycine.
E.   lysine.

16. Potassium depletion causes

A.   extramuscular acidosis.
B.   muscular weakness.
C.   diarrhoea.
D.   cardiac arrhythmias.
E.   renal tubular damage.

17. Doppler ultrasound

A.   is used to monitor fetal breathing.
B.   is used in fetal heart rate monitors.
C.   can be used to measure blood velocity in the fetus.
D.   measures proton relaxation times.
E.   requires injection of contrast agents.

18. The following are structural aberrations of chromosomes:

A.   deletions.
B.   inversions.
C.   aneuploidy.
D.   polyploidy.
E.   translocations.

19. Messenger RNA (mRNA):

A.   synthesis is dependent on RNA polymerase.
B.   is an exact copy of sense DNA.
C.   contains exons.
D.   is measured by Western analysis.
E.   translation occurs in the nucleus.

20. A woman who has a rhesus (Rh) genotype of Cde/CDe

A.   could develop anti-C antibodies.
B.   could safely be transfused with D positive blood.
C.   may develop anti-E antibodies.
D.   should receive anti-D immunoglobulin after giving birth to a Rh (D) positive infant.
E.   is Rh negative.

21. In diseases determined by dominant genes

A. a sibling of an affected person will always be affected.
B. homozygous affected parents will always produce affected offspring.
C. the parents of affected persons have an increased rate of consanguinous marriage.
D. normal children of affected parents have normal offspring.
E. new cases can arise by spontaneous mutation.

22. Autoantibodies are found in

A. systemic lupus erythematosus.
B. rheumatoid arthritis.
C. pernicious anaemia.
D. bronchial asthma.
E. chronic active hepatitis.

23. Concerning immunoglobulins in pregnancy

A. Maternal IgM is responsible for rhesus iso-immunisation in the fetus.
B. The IgA concentration in cord blood is higher than that in maternal blood.
C. IgE crosses the placenta readily.
D. IgG crosses the placenta readily.
E. Fetal IgM is dimeric.

24. The biological effects of complement in the human include

A. opsonisation.
B. cell membrane lysis.
C. participation in the blood coagulation process.
D. promotion of sperm motility.
E. prevention of immune rejection of trophoblast.

25. T lymphocytes

A. differentiate in the thymus.
B. are involved in the generation of both cell-mediated and immoral immune responses.
C. are the predominant lymphoid population in decidua.
D. are the predominant lymphoid population in peripheral blood.
E. are the major cell type in the germinal centres of lymph nodes.

26. Natural killer (NK) cells

A. are related to B cells.
B. have large granular lymphocyte morphology.
C. have receptors for HLA class I molecules.
D. are present in large numbers in decidua during the first trimester.
E. express CD3 (cluster differentiation antigen 3) on their surface.

27. Early blood-borne dissemination is a characteristic feature of

A. carcinoma of the endometrium.
B. osteosarcoma.
C. basal cell carcinoma.
D. carcinoma of the cervix.
E. choriocarcinoma.

28. In tissue pigmentation, the following are associated:

A. kernicterus and conjugated bilirubin.
B. Addison's disease and increased cutaneous melanin.
C. melanosis coli and bile pigments.
D. Wilson's disease and copper deposition in the cornea.
E. corpus luteum and carotenoids.

29. The following cells may be phagocytic:

A. neutrophils.
B. Kupffer cells.
C. monocytes.
D. Hofbauer cells.
E. plasma cells.

30. In healing by primary intention, the following events occur:

A. formation of a fibrin-free haematoma.
B. an acute inflammatory reaction.
C. migration of epithelial cells within 6 hours.
D. phagocytosis.
E. invasion by capillary buds within 3 days.

31. The following are premalignant conditions:

A. diverticular disease of the large bowel.
B. ulcerative colitis.
C. pulmonary asbestosis.

D.   Paget's disease of the bone.
E.   condylomata lata of the vulva.

32. In tumours of bone

A.   primary malignancy is more common than secondary malignancy.
B.   osteoma rarely present in skull bones.
C.   osteosarcoma is associated with Paget's disease of bone.
D.   lymph node metastases are unusual.
E.   simple bone cysts have a strong tendency to recur.

33. In beta thalassaemia

A.   the erythrocytes will sickle at low oxygen tension.
B.   a homozygous fetus is usually anaemic.
C.   stainable iron stores in the marrow are usually decreased.
D.   target cells may be found in the peripheral blood.
E.   erythrocyte survival time is increased.

34. The following are adverse effects of blood transfusion:

A.   hypothermia.
B.   haemoglobinuria.
C.   hypocalcaemia.
D.   hypokalaemia.
E.   thrombocytosis.

35. Bradykinin

A.   causes vasodilatation.
B.   increases vascular permeability.
C.   is formed by the action of kallikrein.
D.   is predominantly inactivated in the lungs.
E.   is metabolised to kininogen.

36. The partial pressure of carbon dioxide in arterial blood may be raised in

A.   residence at high altitude.
B.   gross obesity.
C.   acidaemia due to renal failure.
D.   hyperventilation.
E.   pregnancy.

37. Pain

A. is transmitted along the same pathways in the spinal cord as temperature.
B. arises from the stimulation of free nerve endings.
C. is transmitted in nerves which synapse in spinal ganglia.
D. sensitivity is absent from the parietal peritoneum.
E. fibres from the uterus accompany autonomic nerve fibres.

38. A fall in plasma osmotic pressure

A. is a normal feature of early pregnancy.
B. stimulates vasopressin release.
C. may result in pulmonary oedema.
D. increases thirst.
E. results in a reduction in urine volume.

39. Concerning lecithins:

A. They are polypeptides.
B. Amniotic fluid levels diminish after 33 weeks of pregnancy.
C. Their formation can be inferred from the sphingomyelin level in amniotic fluid.
D. They contain palmitic acid.
E. They act by decreasing surface tension in pulmonary alveoli.

40. Glomerular filtration increases

A. when renal blood flow increases.
B. when plasma oncotic pressure increases.
C. in the remaining kidney following contralateral nephrectomy.
D. following ipsilateral ureteric obstruction.
E. following plasma volume expansion.

41. During the production of urine

A. the proximal renal tubules return about 75% of the water entering them to the blood.
B. the proximal renal tubules present 30–60 litres of water daily to the loops of Henle.
C. the osmotic pressure of the filtrate in the renal cortex is higher than that in the medulla.
D. antidiuretic hormone (ADH) increases the permeability of the walls of the collecting ducts to water.
E. in pregnancy, the glomerular filtration rate decreases.

42. Mast cells

A. normally constitute 3% of circulating leucocytes.
B. are formed in the liver.
C. contain cytoplasmic granules.
D. produce heparin.
E. have receptors for immunoglobulin.

43. The conjugation of bilirubin

A. takes place in hepatocytes.
B. is catalysed by UDP glucuronyl transferase.
C. is inhibited by phenobarbitone.
D. renders it water soluble.
E. is impaired in acute biliary obstruction.

44. Chylomicrons:

A. are synthesised in adipose sites.
B. are a major component of bile.
C. contain triglycerides.
D. are predominantly composed of free fatty acids.
E. are not found in the peripheral circulation.

45. Metabolic acidosis

A. results in an elevation of the plasma bicarbonate concentration.
B. may result from methanol ingestion.
C. stimulates ventilation.
D. decreases the ionised fraction of plasma calcium.
E. results in a fall in urinary pH.

46. During a normal adult cardiac cycle

A. the mitral valve is closed in late diastole.
B. atrial contraction is responsible for 70% of ventricular filling.
C. ventricular ejection slows down as systole progresses.
D. peak right ventricular pressure is less than peak left ventricular pressure during systole.
E. at the end of systole each ventricle contains about 50 ml of blood.

47. In the brachial artery

A. the pulse wave travels to the wrist at the same speed as the arterial blood.
B. the pulse pressure rises with increasing age.
C. the main contribution to systolic blood pressure is skeletal muscle tone.
D. mean pressure rises when the hand is raised above heart level.
E. the pulse pressure is normally about 120 mmHg.

48. The sympathetic nervous system supplies

A. dilator fibres to the bronchial tree.
B. constrictor fibres to the coronary arteries.
C. constrictor fibres to the ciliary muscle.
D. inhibitory fibres to the detrusor muscle.
E. constrictor fibres to the muscles of the small intestine.

49. In the maternal haematological response to pregnancy

A. the total white cell count is increased.
B. the platelet count is increased.
C. the mean red cell haemoglobin concentration is increased.
D. the red cell mass is increased.
E. the reticulocyte count is decreased.

50. During normal pregnancy, the daily urinary excretion of

A. lactose is increased.
B. total amino acids is decreased.
C. total protein is decreased.
D. vitamin B_{12} is increased.
E. folate is decreased.

March 2000 Paper 1

1. The obturator nerve

A. is a branch of the sacral plexus.
B. emerges from the lateral border of the psoas muscle.
C. supplies the pelvic parietal peritoneum.
D. supplies the hip joint.
E. supplies the lateral side of the thigh.

2. The following are sites of anastomosis between systemic and portal veins:

A. lower third of the oesophagus.
B. sigmoid colon.
C. umbilicus.
D. terminal rectum.
E. ureters at the pelvic brim.

3. Concerning the spinal cord and its meninges:

A. The pain pathways run in the posterior columns.
B. The pathways for discriminative touch run in the posterior columns.
C. The cord in the adult terminates at the level of the third lumbar vertebra.
D. The dural sac (lumbar cistern) terminates at the level of the lumbosacral junction.
E. The anterior corticospinal tract carries uncrossed motor fibres.

4. The right ovarian artery

A. arises from the abdominal aorta above the renal artery.
B. passes posterior to the third (horizontal) part of the duodenum.
C. passes posterior to the genitofemoral nerve.
D. supplies the right ureter.
E. anastomoses with the right uterine artery.

5. The ureter

A. is supplied in part by the ovarian artery.
B. lies lateral to the transverse processes of the lumbar vertebrae.
C. passes above the genitofemoral nerve.
D. is lined by a simple columnar epithelium.
E. passes below the uterine artery.

6. Concerning the rectus sheath:

A. Above the costal margin rectus abdominis lies on the costal cartilages.
B. Below the arcuate line the internal oblique splits to enclose rectus abdominis.
C. It contains the musculophrenic artery.
D. It is innervated by the ilioinguinal nerve.
E. Pyramidalis is innervated by the subcostal nerve.

7. The obturator internus muscle

A. leaves the pelvis through the obturator foramen.
B. is inserted onto the greater trochanter of the femur.
C. forms the roof of the ischiorectal fossa.
D. is innervated by the femoral nerve.
E. has a fascia on its pelvic surface which gives origin to the levator ani.

8. Concerning the diaphragm:

A. The vena caval opening lies within the central tendon.
B. It has an aperture for the oesophagus at the level of the 12th thoracic vertebra.
C. It is attached to the pericardium.
D. Motor innervation is received from the lower six intercostal nerves.
E. Sensory innervations are derived solely from the anterior primary rami of the third, fourth and fifth cervical nerves.

9. The external iliac artery

A. enters the thigh anterior to the inguinal ligament.
B. at its origin is crossed by the ureter.
C. at its origin is crossed by the ovarian vessels.
D. lies medial to the external iliac vein at its distal end.
E. gives rise to the deep external pudendal artery.

10. In the femoral triangle, the femoral artery is

A. crossed by the superficial circumflex iliac vein.
B. posterior to the femoral branch of the genitofemoral nerve.
C. medial to the long saphenous vein.
D. posterior to the femoral vein at the apex of the triangle.
E. medial to the femoral nerve.

11. The seminal vesicles

A. contain spermatids.
B. secrete hyaluronidase.
C. secrete acid phosphatase.
D. secrete fructose.
E. secrete prostaglandins.

12. The female urinary bladder

A. is in contact with the supravaginal uterine cervix.
B. is joined to the umbilicus by the urachus.
C. is separated from the posterior surface of the pubis by peritoneum.
D. is connected laterally to the tendinous arch of the pelvic fascia.
E. receives visceral afferent innervation from the pudendal nerve.

13. The ductus venosus

A. is part of the embryonic heart.
B. is a shunt preventing blood from passing to the fetal lungs.
C. gives rise to the ligamentum teres.
D. carries blood with a higher Po_2 than umbilical arterial blood.
E. is derived from the anterior cardinal vein.

14. Concerning gonadal development:

A. The histological appearance of the primitive gonad is similar in both sexes until 42 days after fertilisation.
B. The ovary develops in the medulla of the primitive gonad.
C. The histo-differentiation of the testis begins later than that of the ovary.
D. Primary sex cells (gonocytes) have a haploid number of chromosomes.
E. Mitosis in oogonia is not completed by the end of the first year of life.

15. Trophoblast

A. develops from the blastocyst.
B. gives rise to the fetal blood vessels in the placenta.
C. enters the maternal circulation during normal pregnancy.
D. replaces endothelium of pregnant spiral arterioles.
E. is genetically identical to deciduas.

16. Prolactin

A. release is stimulated by thyrotropin-releasing hormone.
B. plasma levels are raised in the first trimester of pregnancy.
C. is identical to human placental lactogen.
D. controls milk ejection.
E. release is inhibited by metoclopramide.

17. Concerning growth hormone:

A. Plasma levels are reduced by glucose infusion.
B. Maternal plasma levels are directly related to fetal growth.
C. It is active on bone only until the epiphyses fuse.
D. Its secretion is controlled by the hypothalamus.
E. Increased activity produces a positive nitrogen balance.

18. Arginine vasopressin

A. reduces glomerular filtration rate.
B. controls water loss in the proximal renal tubule.
C. is synthesised by the posterior pituitary gland.
D. is released in response to a rise in plasma osmolality.
E. is released in response to a fall in circulating plasma volume.

19. In the human testis

A. the main site of testosterone synthesis is the Sertoli cell.
B. testosterone synthesis is stimulated by follicle stimulating hormone (FSH).
C. the predominant androgen product is androstenedione.
D. the Leydig cells synthesise testosterone.
E. inhibin is synthesised by the Sertoli cell.

20. Actions of insulin include stimulation of

A. glycogenolysis by the liver.
B. cellular uptake of amino acids.
C. entry of glucose into neurones.

D. entry of glucose into adipose tissue.
E. cellular uptake of potassium.

21. Insulin secretion is stimulated by

A. gastrin.
B. noradrenaline (norepinephrine).
C. somatostatin.
D. glucagon.
E. arginine.

22. The following statements about testicular hormones are true:

A. Testosterone reduces plasma luteinising hormone levels.
B. Inhibin increases plasma follicle-stimulating hormone levels.
C. Oestrogens are formed in the testis.
D. Testosterone is excreted in urine as 17-ketosteroids.
E. Testosterone in plasma is partly bound to albumin.

23. Sex hormone-binding globulin

A. levels are increased in pregnancy.
B. is the main binding protein for progesterone.
C. levels are decreased during oestrogen therapy.
D. is the main binding protein for aldosterone.
E. has a greater affinity than albumin for testosterone.

24. The following substances are steroids:

A. aldosterone.
B. follicle-stimulating hormone.
C. vitamin D.
D. inhibin.
E. thyroxine.

25. During pregnancy, the uterine decidua synthesises

A. human chorionic gonadotrophin.
B. prostaglandin E_2.
C. progesterone.
D. prolactin.
E. oxytocin.

26. The actions of growth hormone include

A. promotion of protein synthesis.
B. facilitation of the hepatic synthesis of somatomedin C (insulin-like growth factor).
C. promotion of the insulin-mediated uptake of glucose.
D. stimulation of lipolysis.
E. stimulation of the growth spurt at the onset of puberty.

27. Calcitonin

A. is synthesised in the parathyroid glands.
B. is a decapeptide.
C. secretion is increased at serum calcium levels below 1.5 mmol/1 (6.1 mg/l00 ml).
D. inhibits bone resorption.
E. increases renal tubular excretion of calcium.

28. Vasopressin

A. is a nonapeptide.
B. is synthesised in the posterior pituitary gland.
C. release is increased when plasma osmolality rises.
D. release is increased by haemorrhage.
E. plasma concentration is reduced in pregnancy.

29. Concerning androgens in normal premenopausal women:

A. 95% of circulating testosterone is derived from peripheral conversion of androstenedione.
B. The ovaries and adrenals contribute equally to circulating androgen concentrations.
C. DHEAS (dehydroepiandrosterone sulphate) is derived almost exclusively from the adrenal glands.
D. About 50% of circulating testosterone is bound to sex hormone-binding globulin (SHBG).
E. Testosterone promotes the synthesis of SHBG.

30. Concerning ovarian function:

A. Progesterone is the major steroid of the developing follicle.
B. Granulosa cells secrete oestradiol.
C. Oestradiol is derived from androgen precursors.
D. Insulin-like growth factor (somatomedin C is not secreted by the ovary.
E. Circulating inhibin concentrations are a marker of granulosa cell function.

31. Human chorionic gonadotrophin

A. is a glycoprotein.
B. secretion peaks at 20 weeks of gestation.
C. has intrinsic anti-thyroid activity.
D. is synthesised by the corpus luteum of pregnancy.
E. binds to luteinising hormone (LH) receptors.

32. The following are caused by herpes simplex virus:

A. acute gingivostomatitis.
B. cold sores.
C. cervical warts.
D. meningoencephalitis.
E. shingles.

33. The germination of tetanus spores in a wound is inhibited by

A. tissue trauma.
B. oxygen.
C. injection of anti-toxin.
D. injection of toxoid.
E. removal of devitalised tissue.

34. Cytomegalovirus

A. is an adenovirus.
B. may be cultured readily in cell-free media.
C. is a cause of fetal cerebral calcification.
D. causes haemolytic anaemia in the neonate.
E. may be transmitted in saliva.

35. Concerning rubella

A. it has an incubation period of 7–10 days.
B. recurrent infection is a common cause of congenital malformation.
C. specific antibodies occur within 14 days of infection.
D. individuals are infectious before the appearance of the rash.
E. an attenuated live virus is used in immunisation.

36. Actinomyces israelii

A. is a rickettsia.
B. forms yellow granules in pus.
C. is a commensal in the mouth.

D.   is a commensal in the vagina.
E.   is usually resistant to penicillin.

37. Diseases caused by spirochaetes include

A.   Weil's disease.
B.   lymphogranuloma venereum.
C.   pinta.
D.   Vincent's angina.
E.   Bilharzia.

38. The following antibiotics act on bacterial cell walls:

A.   penicillin.
B.   ceftazidime.
C.   metronidazole.
D.   clindamycin.
E.   gentamicin.

39. Listeria monocytogenes

A.   can grow at 6°C.
B.   is a gut commensal.
C.   is a Gram-negative bacillus.
D.   infection is best treated with benzyl penicillin.
E.   is a cause of septicaemia in neonates.

40. The following antibiotics are usually effective against Pseudomonas aeruginosa

A.   cephradine.*
B.   amoxycillin.
C.   carbenicillin.
D.   gentamicin.
E.   trimethoprim.

41. Metronidazole

A.   is effective against Giardia lamblia.
B.   is effective when administered per rectum.
C.   should not be administered intravenously.
D.   is usually effective against Entamoeba histolytica.
E.   interferes with ethanol metabolism.

---

*   Registered international non-proprietary name is now cefradine; BNF 48, September 2004.

42. The following have an anti-emetic action:

A. hyoscine hydrobromide.
B. morphine sulphate.
C. chlorpropamide.
D. promethazine hydrochloride.
E. perphenazine.

43. Beta sympathomimetic drugs may

A. cause bronchospasm.
B. reduce the frequency of uterine contractions.
C. cause heart block.
D. reduce diastolic blood pressure.
E. increase blood glucose concentration.

44. The following substances are sympathomimetic amines:

A. amphetamines.
B. ephedrine.
C. histamine.
D. isoprenaline.
E. chlorpromazine.

45. The following drugs can cause bronchoconstriction

A. propranolol.
B. atropine.
C. morphine.
D. ritodrine.
E. aspirin.

46. The following drugs have anticholinergic effects:

A. propantheline bromide.
B. carbachol.
C. distigmine bromide.
D. benzhexol.
E. atropine.

47. Thiopentone sodium administered intravenously

A. is a potent muscle relaxant.
B. is predominantly excreted by the kidney.
C. binds to protein.

D.   is fat soluble.
E.   crosses the placenta.

48. Hypokalaemia may be caused by

A.   bendrofluazide.*
B.   digoxin.
C.   spironolactone.
D.   carbenoxolone.
E.   amiloride.

49. The following statistical statements are correct:

A.   In the normal distribution, the value of the mode is 1.73 x that of the median.
B.   In a distribution skewed to the right, the mean lies to the left of the median.
C.   In the series: 2;7;5;2;3;2;5;8, the mode is 2.
D.   Student's t-test is designed to correct for skewed distribution.
E.   The Chi-squared test may be used when data are not normally distributed.

50. In a randomised double-blind trial comparing a new drug with a placebo

A.   the patients will be taking either of two active drugs.
B.   patients can choose their method of treatment.
C.   doctors prescribing treatment decide which patients take the new drug.
D.   a large trial is more likely to give a statistically significant result than a small trial.
E.   half of the patients will take the new drug.

*   Registered international non-proprietary name is now bendromefluazide; BNF 48, September 2004.

March 2000
Paper 2

1. Concerning pH:

A. In blood, pH is regulated predominantly by bicarbonate.
B. The higher the pH, the higher the hydrogen ion concentration.
C. The pH of gastric juice is 5.5.
D. The pH of urine decreases after the ingestion of ammonium chloride.
E. The pH inside cells is higher than that in plasma.

2. In the adrenal cortex

A. ACTH controls the hydroxylation of cholesterol to pregnenolone.
B. oestradiol can be formed from testosterone.
C. androstenedione and testosterone are interconvertible.
D. 17α-hydroxyprogesterone is a breakthrough product of corticosterone.
E. aldosterone is formed from corticosterone.

3. The conversion of glucose to lactic acid

A. occurs in a single enzymatic reaction.
B. is the only pathway for the synthesis of ATP in the red blood cell.
C. is a reversible process in skeletal muscle.
D. is inhibited by high cellular concentrations of ATP.
E. occurs in skeletal muscle when the availability of oxygen is limited.

4. Glucagon

A. is a polypeptide hormone.
B. is secreted by the beta cells of the pancreatic islets.
C. causes muscle glycogenolysis.
D. has a half-life of 5–10 minutes in the circulation.
E. secretion is stimulated by cortisol.

5. Concerning prostaglandins (PG)

A. Arachidonic acid is the precursor for PG biosynthesis.
B. PG synthetase (cyclooxygenase) catalyses arachidonic acid conversion to PG endoperoxides.
C. Nonsteroidal anti-inflammatory drugs inhibit PG dehydrogenase.
D. Mefenamic acid is a more potent inhibitor of PG synthesis than aspirin.
E. $PGF_{2\alpha}$ is excreted unchanged in urine.

6. Amniotic fluid

A. at term is hyperosmolar compared to fetal plasma.
B. normally contains maternal and fetal cells.
C. contains a higher concentration of α-fetoprotein (AFP) at 16 weeks than at term.
D. contains bilirubin.
E. contains phospholipids.

7. Oestradiol

A. is formed by aromatisation of testosterone.
B. does not bind to albumin.
C. is formed in tissues other than the ovaries.
D. is the most abundant oestrogen in late pregnancy.
E. binds to a specific cell surface receptor.

8. 2,3-diphosphoglycerate (2,3-DPG)

A. is present at higher concentrations in maternal erythrocytes than fetal erythrocytes.
B. binds more avidly to haemoglobin A than to haemoglobin F.
C. increases the affinity of haemoglobin for oxygen.
D. is a phospholipid.
E. is synthesised by the pentose phosphate pathway.

9. Ethanol

A. consumed in excess stimulates fatty acid oxidation.
B. suppresses arginine vasopressin secretion.
C. promotes gluconeogenesis.
D. is oxidised to acetaldehyde.
E. is metabolised predominantly by the liver.

10. Glucocorticoids

A. promote hepatic gluconeogenesis.
B. suppress uptake of glucose by muscles.
C. promote protein breakdown.
D. promote fat breakdown.
E. increase glycolysis in adipose tissue.

11. Fibrinogen

A. levels are usually low during pregnancy.
B. is a substrate for thrombin.
C. at elevated plasma levels causes a reduction in the erythrocyte sedimentation rate (ESR).
D. is synthesised in the liver.
E. is a Bence Jones' protein.

12. Concerning maternal-fetal placental transfer

A. Oxygen transfer is facilitated by the fetal oxygen dissociation curve being to the right of that of the mother.
B. Bicarbonate ions diffuse across the placenta more easily than carbon dioxide.
C. Glucose is transferred by simple diffusion.
D. Immunoglobulin G crosses the placenta.
E. The placenta is impermeable to maternal ketone bodies.

13. Vitamin K

A. is synthesised by bacteria.
B. is stored in large quantities in the liver.
C. is necessary for the synthesis of factor VII.
D. is necessary for the synthesis of factor IX.
E. deficiency causes hypothrombinaemia.

14. Plasma concentrations of the following substances are typically raised in pregnancy

A. caeruloplasmin.
B. albumin.
C. vitamin B_{12}.
D. urea.
E. pituitary gonadotrophins.

15. In one turn of the tricarboxylic acid cycle

A. three molecules of carbon dioxide (CO_2) are produced.
B. reduced nicotinamide adenine dinucleotide (NADH) are produced.
C. reduced dihydroflavine adenine dinucleotide ($FADH_2$) are produced.
D. guanosine triphosphate (GTP) is produced.
E. acetyl coenzyme A (Acetyl CoA) is used.

16. Lactose

A. is a non-reducing sugar.
B. may be detected in the urine of a normal pregnant woman.
C. is a major constituent of seminal fluid.
D. is galactosyl-glucose.
E. is catabolised by the liver.

17. Plasma low-density lipoproteins (LDL)

A. are less dense than chylomicrons.
B. predominantly contain non-esterified fatty acids.
C. are the main source of cholesterol for steroid synthesis.
D. contain more protein by dry weight than high density lipoproteins.
E. attach to specific cell membrane receptors.

18. The ultrasound energy used in a real-time machine for diagnostic imaging

A. is pulsed.
B. has a velocity measured in metres per second.
C. has a velocity which is the same in all human tissues.
D. has a frequency measured in decibels.
E. is entirely dissipated within the tissues.

19. In the human

A. haploid cells contain homologous pairs of chromosomes.
B. polyploid cells contain extra sets of chromosomes.
C. monosomic cells contain an extra chromosome.
D. haploid cells contain 22 autosomes.
E. chromosomes divide during the S phase of the cell cycle.

20. The following are inherited as autosomal recessive conditions

A. tuberous sclerosis.
B. phenylketonuria.
C. achondroplasia.

D.   sickle cell anaemia.

E.   Von Gierke's disease.

21. Chromosomes

A.   are found in the same number in all mammalian cells.

B.   can be analysed more quickly from a blood sample than from an amniotic fluid sample.

C.   can be reliably identified by their lengths.

D.   the Y chromosome is larger than the X chromosome.

E.   DNA content is doubled during the S (synthesis) phase of the cell cycle.

22. In DNA

A.   a codon is a sequence of three bases.

B.   all codons have an identified function.

C.   there is a greater variety of amino acids than there are different codons.

D.   replication can be initiated at several different points along a chromosome.

E.   complementary pairing precedes messenger RNA synthesis.

23. Type III (immune complex-related) hypersensitivity is characterised by

A.   damage localised to a particular cell type.

B.   decreased vascular permeability.

C.   microthrombus formation.

D.   complement activation.

E.   mediation by IgE antibodies.

24. Steps involved in the identification of restriction fragment length polymorphisms (RFLP) include

A.   Western blotting.

B.   restriction enzyme digestion.

C.   Southern blotting.

D.   agarose gel electrophoresis.

E.   thin layer chromatography.

25. The following are causes of hypokalaemia:

A.   angiotensin-converting enzyme (ACE) inhibitors.

B.   Addison's disease.

C. diarrhoea.
D. digoxin overdose.
E. metabolic alkalosis.

26. Features of disseminated intravascular coagulation include

A. thrombocythaemia.
B. petechiae.
C. haemorrhage.
D. reduced circulating fibrin degradation products.
E. small-vessel thrombosis.

27. Granulation tissue contains the following

A. elastin fibres.
B. inflammatory cells.
C. capillaries.
D. epithelioid cells.
E. fibroblasts.

28. In sarcoidosis,

A. lesions are confined to the lung.
B. the Mantoux test is strongly positive.
C. caseation is not present.
D. the lesions contain giant cells.
E. the Kveim test is a useful adjunct to diagnosis.

29. Wound healing is delayed by

A. insulin.
B. ultraviolet light.
C. zinc deficiency.
D. low temperature.
E. glucocorticosteroids.

30. Adenocarcinoma is the commonest type of primary malignant tumour to occur in the

A. bladder.
B. lung.
C. oesophagus.
D. fallopian tube.
E. testis.

31. The following provide conclusive evidence of pregnancy in uterine curettings:

A. decidua compacta.
B. Arias-Stella changes in endometrial glands.
C. spiral arterioles.
D. plasma cell infiltration.
E. chorionic villi.

32. The parathyroid glands

A. originate from the pharyngeal cleft ectoderm.
B. secrete parathyroid hormone via the chief (principal) cells.
C. secrete calcitonin via the oxyphyl cells.
D. may become hyperplastic in the presence of intestinal malabsorption.
E. may develop adenomas in association with islet cell tumours of the pancreas.

33. Complications of myocardial infarction include

A. fibrinous pericarditis.
B. aortic aneurysm.
C. ventricular mural thrombi.
D. coronary atherosclerosis.
E. ventricular aneurysm.

34. Granulomatous inflammation occurs in

A. lobar pneumonia.
B. pulmonary tuberculosis.
C. sarcoidosis.
D. staphylococcal infection.
E. temporal arteritis.

35. The concentration of urine

A. is due to passive reabsorption of water.
B. is completed in the loop of Henle.
C. occurs progressively along the proximal tubule.
D. is dependent upon arginine vasopressin.
E. is related to the osmolarity of the interstitial fluid of the renal medulla.

36. Concerning haematological changes daring normal pregnancy:

A. Plasma volume increases.
B. The red cell mass decreases.
C. Erythrocyte sedimentation rate is increased.
D. Mean cell volume decreases.
E. Total iron binding capacity increases.

37. Myometrial contractility

A. is calcium-dependent.
B. is associated with phosphorylation of myosin light chain.
C. is independent of cyclic adenosine monophosphate (AMP).
D. is mediated by somatic nerves.
E. depends on myometrial gap junctions.

38. Brown adipose tissue in the human infant is

A. more vascular than normal adipose tissue.
B. a site of heat production.
C. found predominantly in the abdominal wall.
D. innervated.
E. deficient in mitochondria.

39. Angiotensin II

A. is a vasoconstrictor.
B. decreases aldosterone production.
C. is formed mainly in the lungs.
D. is a decapeptide.
E. is produced when the circulating blood volume is reduced.

40. A reduced arterial Pco2

A. occurs in normal pregnancy.
B. occurs at altitudes over 2500 metres.
C. increases cerebral blood flow.
D. leads to a more alkaline urine.
E. reduces blood pH.

41. Gastrointestinal absorption of

A. dietary glucose depends upon intact pancreatic function.
B. vitamin B_{12} requires gastric acid.
C. fats is accomplished by the transport of chylomicrons from the intestinal lumen.

D. iron may be reduced by vitamin C administration.
E. unhydrolised polysaccharides does not occur.

42. Mast cells

A. normally form 3% of circulating leukocytes.
B. release histamine on degranulation.
C. contain heparin.
D. control melanin formation in the epidermis.
E. have a specific affinity for antibody of the IgA class.

43. Characteristic features of Addisonian pernicious anaemia are:

A. leucocytosis.
B. inheritance as an autosomal dominant trait.
C. a raised mean corpuscular haemoglobin concentration.
D. an increased incidence of gastric neoplasia.
E. an increased incidence of primary hypothyroidism.

44. The events in normal micturition in women include

A. contraction of the perineal muscles.
B. initial relaxation of the detrusor muscle.
C. a constant increase in intra-abdominal pressure.
D. no change in intravesical pressure.
E. urinary flow of a maximum of 5 ml per second.

45. The following may occur in uncomplicated haemolytic jaundice

A. bilirubinuria.
B. high serum levels of conjugated bilirubin.
C. urobilinuria.
D. high serum levels of alkaline phosphatase.
E. reticulocytosis.

46. During the normal cell cycle

A. the principal phase of deoxyribonucleic acid (DNA) synthesis is G_1.
B. a tetraploid quantity of DNA is present at the end of G_2.
C. G_2 is the post-mitotic resting phase.
D. cells are generally sensitive to anti-metabolites in the S phase.
E. the DNA is completely replicated several times.

47. In the fetal circulation

A. most of the blood from the superior vena cava passes directly from the right to the left atrium.
B. the output of the right ventricle is greater than that of the left.
C. blood in the ascending aorta is more oxygenated than that in the descending aorta.
D. blood in the right ventricle is more oxygenated than blood in the left ventricle.
E. blood in the ductus arteriosus and the right atrium is equally oxygenated.

48. The adult oxygen–haemoglobin dissociation curve is shifted to the left by

A. low temperature.
B. low haemoglobin levels.
C. high altitude.
D. 2,3-diphosphoglyceride.
E. alkalosis.

49. In a healthy woman, renin

A. is secreted only by the kidney.
B. concentration is greater than in the nonpregnant state.
C. concentration is increased by diuretic therapy.
D. converts angiotensinogen into angiotensin II.
E. activity is blocked by captopril.

50. In the small intestine the following substances are absorbed by active processes:

A. water.
B. sodium.
C. vitamin K.
D. amino acids.
E. chloride.

September 2000 Paper 1

1. The internal pudendal artery

A. leaves the pelvis through the lesser sciatic foramen.
B. lies on the medial wall of the ischiorectal fossa.
C. has a branch which pierces the perineal membrane.
D. gives rise to the middle rectal artery.
E. supplies the upper vagina.

2. The obturator artery

A. branches from the posterior trunk of the internal iliac artery.
B. passes through the greater sciatic foramen.
C. is crossed by the ureter.
D. supplies the hip joint.
E. may be replaced by a branch of the superior epigastric artery.

3. The adult pituitary gland

A. contains the paraventricular nuclei.
B. is related to the sphenoid bone.
C. lies inferior to the optic chiasma.
D. contains a pars tuberalis inferiorly.
E. is entirely ectodermal in origin.

4. The following statements about the adrenal glands are correct:

A. The adrenal glands are anterior to the diaphragm.
B. The right adrenal vein drains directly into the inferior vena cava.
C. The lymphatic drainage is to the superficial inguinal nodes.
D. The adrenal cortex contains chromaffin cells.
E. The adrenal medulla develops from mesoderm.

5. The anal canal

A. has an upper part which is innervated by the inferior hypogastric plexus.
B. has a lower part which is supplied by the superior rectal artery.
C. drains lymph to the superficial inguinal nodes from its upper part.
D. has its internal sphincter innervated by the inferior rectal nerve.
E. has a superficial part of its external sphincter attached to the coccyx.

6. The obturator nerve

A. emerges from the lateral border of psoas.
B. is formed from the posterior divisions of the second, third and fourth lumbar nerves.
C. passes lateral to the internal iliac vessels.
D. lies below the obturator artery in the obturator foramen.
E. is separated from the normally sited ovary only by the pelvic peritoneum.

7. The hypothalamus

A. forms part of the mid-brain.
B. is closely related to the optic chiasma.
C. contains the paraventricular nuclei.
D. is a centre for appetite control.
E. has nerve connections with the anterior lobe of the pituitary gland.

8. The ampulla of the fallopian tube

A. is the longest portion of the tube.
B. is developed from the paramesonephric duct.
C. has complex folding of the mucosa.
D. is lined exclusively by ciliated columnar epithelium.
E. has an internal longitudinal muscle coat.

9. In the inguinal canal,

A. the iliohypogastric nerve passes through the canal.
B. the inferior epigastric artery lies at the lateral boundary of the deep inguinal ring.
C. the medial umbilical ligament crosses deep to the posterior wall.
D. the roof is formed by the external oblique muscle.
E. the posterior wall is reinforced medially by the conjoint tendon.

10. The pudendal nerve

A. contains fibres from the first sacral nerve.
B. lies lateral to the internal pudendal artery as it exits from the pelvis.
C. contains sensory fibres from the lower vagina.
D. contains sensory fibres from the skin of the labium majus.
E. innervates obturator internus.

11. The following are derived from the urogenital sinus:

A. the bladder trigone.
B. the ureters.
C. the female urethra.
D. greater vestibular glands.
E. paraurethral glands.

12. In the fetal circulation

A. the ductus venosus delivers blood directly into the superior vena cava.
B. the umbilical artery returns blood from the placenta.
C. the ductus arteriosus carries blood to the lungs.
D. blood returning from the lungs is 90% saturated with oxygen.
E. blood from the inferior vena cava is largely directed through the foramen ovale.

13. Following fertilisation in the human

A. the first polar body is formed.
B. the first cleavage division occurs within 12 hours.
C. the zona pellucida is shed at the second cleavage division.
D. cleavage divisions are mitotic.
E. the mean cell volume decreases with each cleavage division.

14. Parathyroid hormone

A. is a polypeptide.
B. increases bone resorption.
C. decreases phosphate excretion in the urine.
D. secretion is diminished by an increase in serum ionised calcium concentration.
E. decreases the formation of 1,25-dihydroxycholecalciferol.

15. In the renin-angiotensin system

A. renin is an enzyme.
B. angiotensin II is converted to angiotensin I.
C. angiotensinogen is a globulin.
D. renin release is inhibited by sodium restriction.
E. renin is present in amniotic fluid.

16. Concerning thyroid function:

A. thyroid-binding globulin is found entirely within the thyroid gland.
B. triiodothyronine is mainly in the free form in the circulation.
C. triiodothyronine acts more rapidly than thyroxine.
D. a fall in thyroid-binding globulin causes hypothyroidism.
E. thyroxine is a major precursor of triiodothyronine.

17. Thyroxine

A. exists in the free state in the thyroid gland.
B. is more than 99% protein-bound in plasma.
C. is released by the fetal thyroid.
D. in the unbound state in plasma is approximately equal in concentration to unbound triiodothyronine.
E. is actively transported across the placenta.

18. Recognised features of congenital adrenal hyperplasia in the female are:

A. acute hypotension.
B. enlargement of the clitoris.
C. abnormal karyotype.
D. hirsutism.
E. absent uterus.

19. Concerning sex hormones:

A. The ovary secretes androstenedione.
B. The ovary secretes testosterone.
C. The ovary secretes dihydrotestosterone.
D. Sex hormone-binding globulin (SHBG) concentrations are higher in women than in men.
E. Androgens bound to protein have high biological activity.

20. Adrenal androgens

A. are synthesised in the zona glomerulosa of the adrenal cortex.
B. are secreted in excessive amounts in the presence of 11β-hydroxylase deficiency.
C. stimulate protein synthesis.
D. consist mainly of testosterone.
E. are secreted in increased amounts in response to a rise in adrenocorticotrophic hormone.

21. After the menopause

A. the plasma concentration of follicle-stimulating hormone (FSH) increases.
B. the plasma progesterone concentration increases.
C. oestrone is the oestrogen found in highest concentration in the plasma.
D. the plasma testosterone concentration increases.
E. the plasma prolactin concentration increases.

22. Serum concentrations of the following increase during pregnancy:

A. sex hormone-binding globulin.
B. prolactin.
C. total thyroxine.
D. follicle-stimulating hormone.
E. corticotrophin-releasing hormone.

23. The release of catecholamines from the adrenal medulla increases

A. during sleep in healthy individuals.
B. when the nerves to the adrenal gland are stimulated.
C. following an increase in blood sugar.
D. immediately following a myocardial infarction.
E. during acute haemorrhage.

24. Human chorionic gonadotrophin

A. is not produced by the decidua.
B. is biochemically indistinguishable from luteinising hormone.
C. is active if given to nonpregnant women.
D. production rises steadily throughout pregnancy.
E. has no influence upon the production of oestrogens by the placenta.

25. Human placental lactogen

A. concentration in maternal plasma is directly proportional to the functional mass of the placenta.
B. has a half-life in blood of less than one hour.
C. is a steroid hormone.
D. increases the mobilisation of maternal free fatty acids.
E. reaches the same concentration in fetal blood as in maternal blood at term.

26. The secretion of growth hormone

A. occurs in the hypothalamus.
B. ceases when the adult state is reached.
C. is decreased during stress.
D. is increased during fasting.
E. is increased with exercise.

27. Arginine vasopressin

A. is produced in the hypothalamus.
B. is a polypeptide.
C. is structurally similar to prolactin.
D. controls water reabsorption by the kidney.
E. decreases glomerular filtration.

28. Oxytocin

A. is released episodically.
B. causes decreased renal tubular reabsorption of water.
C. is responsible for milk ejection.
D. reduces intestinal peristalsis.
E. inhibits prolactin secretion.

29. The following agents cause myometrial contractions:

A. magnesium sulphate.
B. nifedipine.
C. progesterone.
D. salbutamol.
E. sodium nitroprusside.

30. Renin

A. is secreted by the zona glomerulosa of the adrenal cortex.
B. is a proteolytic enzyme.

C. is secreted at an increased rate if the renal perfusion pressure falls.
D. acts upon circulating angiotensinogen.
E. is released in response to an increase in extracellular fluid volume.

31. Concerning viruses:

A. The core of every virus contains RNA.
B. They usually produce intracellular toxins causing cell death.
C. Antibodies are directed against capsular proteins.
D. They can only be grown in intact cells.
E. Interferons are synthetic antiviral substances.

32. The following organisms are Gram-positive:

A. *Streptococcus pneumoniae.*
B. *Neisseria gonorrhoeae.*
C. *Salmonella typhi.*
D. *Lactobacillus.*
E. *Pseudomonas aeruginosa.*

33. Leptospirosis

A. is caused by a Gram-negative coccobacillus.
B. is frequently transmitted to man from inanimate objects.
C. can result in a severe form of jaundice.
D. is a sexually transmitted disease.
E. is transmitted in pasteurised cow's milk.

34. The following disorders and organisms are correctly paired:

A. ophthalmia neonatorum : *Chlamydia trachomatis.*
B. chancroid : *Haemophilus ducreyii.*
C. sleeping sickness : *Leishmania donovani.*
D. ring worm : *Trichinella spiralis.*
E. non-specific urethritis : *Toxoplasma gondii.*

35. *Candida albicans*

A. is Gram-positive.
B. is a commensal in the bowel.
C. is sensitive to miconazole.
D. causes secondary infection after treatment with broad-spectrum antibiotics.
E. is cultured on alkaline media.

36. Concerning hepatitis B virus infection:

A. Vertical transmission does not occur.
B. Sexual transmission occurs.
C. Core antigenaemia indicates high infectivity.
D. Hepatocellular carcinoma is a recognised complication.
E. An effective vaccine is available.

37. *Pseudomonas aeruginosa*

A. is non-motile.
B. is Gram-positive.
C. does not grow anaerobically.
D. ferments lactose.
E. produces pigment.

38. Oestrogen therapy raises the plasma concentrations of

A. thyroxine-binding globulin.
B. free cortisol.
C. transferrin.
D. albumin.
E. folate.

39. The following agents are bronchodilators:

A. salbutamol.
B. atenolol.
C. prostaglandin F_{2a}.
D. morphine.
E. prednisolone.

40. Subcutaneous atropine injection characteristically produces

A. an increase in heart rate.
B. an increase in salivation.
C. constriction of the pupil.
D. an hypnotic effect.
E. decreased bronchiolar secretion.

41. Concerning heparins:

A. Heparin is synthesised in the lungs.
B. Antithrombin III is necessary for standard heparins to exert their anticoagulant effect.
C. Factor X is inhibited by low-molecular-weight heparins.

D. Low-molecular-weight heparins have a longer half-life than standard heparins.
E. Penicillins potentiate the action of low-molecular-weight heparins.

42. The following substances exert their diuretic actions upon the distal convoluted tubule:

A. bendrofluaside.*
B. fusemide.**
C. bumetanide.
D. mannitol.
E. alcohol.

43. Clomifene citrate

A. is an anti-androgen.
B. does not stimulate ovulation directly.
C. can produce visual disturbances.
D. is generally prescribed throughout the proliferative phase of the menstrual cycle.
E. in the treatment of anovulation, increases the risk of multiple pregnancy.

44. The therapeutic effect of the first drug is enhanced by the second drug:

A. phenytoin – ethinyloestradiol.
B. bromocryptine – metoclopramide.
C. penicillin – probenecid.
D. ritodrine – dexamethasone.
E. warfarin – phenobarbitone.

45. The following cytotoxic drugs are correctly classified:

A. methotrexate: alkylating agent.
B. cyclophosphamide : alkylating agent.
C. vinblastine : antimetabolite.
D. mercaptopurine: antimetabolite.
E. fluorouracil : antibiotic.

46. Halothane produces

A. cardiac arrhythmias.
B. explosive mixtures with air.

---

* Registered international non-proprietary name is bendoflumethiazide; BNF 48, September 2004.
** Registered international non-proprietary name is furosemide; BNF 48, September 2004.

C. liver damage if given repeatedly.
D. myometrial relaxation.
E. bronchial irritation.

47. In a sample of 1000 children, the birth weight was normally distributed with a mean of 3.5 kg and a standard deviation of 700 g.

A. Fifteen infants would be below the fifth centile for weight.
B. The standard error of the birth weight would be about 22 g.
C. The 95th centile for birth weight would be 4.2 kg.
D. No baby would weigh less than 1.4 kg.
E. The median birth weight would be about 3.5 kg.

48. If a distribution of results is markedly skewed to the left

A. the mean is the same as the 50th centile.
B. the same number of values lies on either side of the median.
C. the mode is equal to the median.
D. the Student's t test should be used to compare this distribution with another.
E. logarithmic transformation of the results will produce a distribution closer to the normal.

49. In the statistical analysis of any group of numerical observations

A. the mean is always less than the mode.
B. the median value always lies at the mid-point of the range.
C. standard deviation is always greater than the standard error of the mean.
D. the standard error of the mean is independent of the total number of observations.
E. there are the same number of observations greater than and less than the median value.

50. In a trial of oral hypolycaemic agents, 42 patients were given drug A and 38 drug B. Blood glucose concentrations were measured before and after a single dose of the drug. Drug B apparently caused a greater fall in blood glucose concentration ($P = 0.06$).

A. These results reach an accepted level of statistical significance.
B. Non-parametric statistical analysis should be used if data are not normally distributed.

C. In biological terms, drugs A and B have been shown to be equally effective.
D. 6% more patients responded to drug A than drug B.
E. Unequal numbers in the two groups invalidate the trial.

September 2000 Paper 2

1. The oxidation of pyruvate to carbon dioxide

A. occurs exclusively in the mitochondria of the cell.
B. can occur under anaerobic conditions.
C. involves intermediates which are also involved in amino acid catabolism.
D. is regulated by the concentration of acetyl coenzyme A in the cell.
E. is impaired in thiamine deficiency states.

2. Enzyme activity can be modified by

A. concentration of substrate.
B. concentration of product.
C. pH.
D. temperature.
E. concentration of coenzymes.

3. The rate of transfer of a substance into a cell by active transport

A. may be unrelated to concentration gradient.
B. is dependent upon molecular size.
C. is temperature dependent.
D. has a fixed upper limit.
E. is not reduced by the presence of a structurally similar substance.

4. Fatty acids reaching the liver from the fat stores may be

A. converted to glucose.
B. conjugated with sulphate.
C. metabolised in the tricarboxylic acid cycle.
D. incorporated into endogenous triglyceride.
E. converted into ketones.

5. Concerning folic acid:

A. It is a water soluble vitamin.
B. Conversion of dihydrofolate to tetrahydrofolate is inhibited by methotrexate.
C. Red cell folate concentration can be reduced by phenytoin.
D. Tetrahydrofolic acid is a carrier of 1-carbon units.
E. It is involved in synthesis of purines.

6. Effects of insulin include

A. increase in cellular growth.
B. increased hepatic glycogen synthesis.
C. decreased glycogen synthesis in muscle.
D. increased uptake of potassium ions in muscle.
E. increased uptake of potassium ions in adipose tissue.

7. Surfactant

A. is a carbohydrate.
B. contains significant amounts of 2,3-diphosphoglycerate.
C. is produced by type II alveolar epithelial cells.
D. is present in the fetal lung at 24 weeks of gestation.
E. production in the fetus is increased by glucocorticoids.

8. Histamine

A. is identical to bradykinin.
B. is a derivative of histidine.
C. increases capillary permeability.
D. promotes gastric acid secretion.
E. inhibits the secretion of pepsin.

9. Cholesterol is

A. synthesised in the liver.
B. a C-19 compound.
C. synthesised from acetate.
D. a major constituent of high-density lipoproteins.
E. predominantly excreted unchanged in the urine.

10. Vitamin K is involved in the formation of

A. fibrinogen.
B. factor VIII.

C. factor IX.
D. prothrombin.
E. heparin.

11. Plasma albumin binds the following

A. free fatty acids.
B. triglycerides.
C. oestradiol.
D. bilirubin.
E. iron ions.

12. Within 48 hours of a major surgical operation there is an increase in

A. adrenocorticotrophin secretion.
B. aldosterone secretion.
C. arginine vasopressin secretion.
D. sodium excretion.
E. potassium excretion.

13. Metabolic acidosis

A. can result from potassium deficiency.
B. can result from excess consumption of sodium bicarbonate.
C. leads to an alteration in plasma bicarbonate levels.
D. occurs after the administration of ammonium chloride.
E. can be caused by persistent vomiting.

14. Conjugated bilirubin

A. is produced from haemoglobin.
B. is a constituent of the amniotic fluid in the second trimester.
C. is lipid soluble.
D. is conjugated by the action of alkaline phosphatase.
E. has a normal blood level of about 500 mg/l.

15. Ribonucleic acid (RNA)

A. contains deoxyribose.
B. is composed of two nucleotide units.
C. is the main constituent of chromosomes.
D. is the main constituent of ribosomes.
E. is required during protein synthesis.

16. Alkalosis can be caused by

A. excessive vomiting.
B. cardiac failure.
C. hyperventilation.
D. hyperaldosteronism.
E. therapeutic doses of magnesium trisilicate.

17. Concerning radiotherapy:

A. A gray (100 rads) is a unit of energy absorption.
B. Liver parenchyma is more radiosensitive than intestinal epithelium.
C. Cells with a slow reproductive capacity are usually the most radiosensitive.
D. The concentration of intracellular oxygen is inversely proportional to the susceptibility of the cell to radiation damage.
E. Well-differentiated tumours show higher radiosensitivity than anaplastic tumours.

18. The following disorders have an X-linked pattern of inheritance:

A. glucose-6-phosphate dehydrogenase deficiency.
B. Kleinfelter syndrome.
C. adrenogenital syndrome.
D. haemophilia B.
E. familial hypercholesterolaemia.

19. In the female

A. only the X chromosome of maternal origin is active.
B. the Barr body is sex chromatin.
C. about 80% of polymorphonuclear leucocytes have a 'drumstick' of chromatin.
D. an extra X chromosome is associated with two Barr bodies.
E. an extra X chromosome is associated with below average intelligence.

20. The following statements relate to familial diseases:

A. Achondroplasia is a dominant trait.
B. Babies with Down syndrome usually have 46 chromosomes.
C. Congenital pyloric stenosis is commoner in babies of affected parents than in the general population.
D. All the daughters of a female carrier of red green colour blindness are themselves carriers.
E. Haemophilia occurs in all the sons of an affected father.

21. The following genetic disorders are inherited as autosomal recessives:

A. Duchenne muscular dystrophy.
B. Huntingdon's chorea.
C. Tay-Sach's disease.
D. retinoblastoma.
E. achondroplasia.

22. The following are structural abnormalities of chromosomes:

A. deletions.
B. duplications.
C. aneuploidy.
D. polyploidy.
E. translocations.

23. Concerning immunoglobulins:

A. IgG contains two heavy chains.
B. IgM is produced before IgG in the immune response.
C. IgE is the principal immunoglobulin secreted by mucous membranes.
D. IgA is the principal immunoglobulin involved in allergic reactions.
E. IgA is secreted in breast milk.

24. B lymphocytes may

A. produce tumour necrosis factor.
B. produce complement.
C. present antigens to T cells.
D. contribute to delayed hypersensitivity.
E. produce IgE.

25. Antibodies play an important part in the development of

A. phagocytosis.
B. the Mantoux response.
C. erythroblastosis fetalis.
D. hyperemesis gravidarum.
E. anaphylaxis.

26. The following agents are correctly paired with the named tumours:

A. androgenic steroids : vaginal clear cell adenocarcinoma.
B. aflatoxins : liver cell carcinoma.

C. β-naphthylamine : bronchial carcinoma.
D. asbestos: peritoneal mesothelioma.
E. vinyl chloride : hepatic angiosarcoma.

27. The following are examples of type-III hypersensitivity (immune-complex) diseases:

A. autoimmune haemolytic anaemia.
B. systemic lupus erythematosus.
C. glomerulonephritis.
D. tuberculosis.
E. sarcoidosis.

28. Chemical mediators concerned in the production of an inflammatory response include

A. 5-hydroxytryptamine.
B. aldosterone.
C. glucocorticoids.
D. bradykinin.
E. leukotrienes.

29. In cystic fibrosis, abnormalities are seen in the

A. pancreas.
B. salivary glands.
C. brain.
D. kidneys.
E. ileum.

30. Immunodeficiency states may be associated with

A. viral infection of T lymphocytes.
B. B cell lymphomas.
C. glucocorticoid administration.
D. haemolytic disease of the newborn.
E. untreated Hodgkin's lymphoma.

31. The following statements relate to embryonic tumours:

A. An ovarian teratoma is usually malignant.
B. A nephroblastoma may be benign.
C. A neuroblastoma can arise in the adrenal medulla.
D. A hamartoma is usually malignant.
E. Choriocarcinoma may arise in a teratoma.

32. The parathyroid glands

A. originate from the pharyngeal cleft ectoderm.
B. secrete parathyroid hormone via the chief cells.
C. secrete calcitonin via the oxyphil cells.
D. may become hyperplastic in the presence of intestinal malabsorption.
E. may develop adenomas in association with islet cell tumours of the pancreas.

33. The following conditions may lead to hydronephrosis:

A. mercury poisoning.
B. cervical carcinoma.
C. renal calculi.
D. renal vein thrombosis.
E. posterior urethral valves.

34. The following changes in ventilation occur during pregnancy:

A. a decrease in respiratory rate.
B. a decrease in Pco_2.
C. a decrease in residual volume.
D. an increase in tidal volume.
E. an increase in Po_2.

35. The following are required for haemostatic clot formation:

A. conversion of prothrombin to thrombin.
B. platelet phospholipids.
C. active conversion of plasminogen to plasmin.
D. fibrin degradation products.
E. antithrombin.

36. In the human neonate, compared with the adult

A. the liver has less ability to conjugate bilirubin.
B. the blood–brain barrier is less permeable to bilirubin.
C. heat regulation is more efficient.
D. red blood cells have greater affinity for oxygen.
E. the haemoglobin concentration is greater.

37. In the cardiac cycle of a healthy adult at rest

A. the stroke volume is about 70 ml.
B. the duration of ventricular systole is about ten times as long as that of ventricular diastole.

C. the first heart sound corresponds to the closure of the atrioventricular valves.
D. the apex beat can be felt in the seventh intercostal space.
E. the contraction is initiated by the atrioventricular node.

38. 2,3-diphosphoglycerate

A. is present at higher concentrations in maternal erythrocytes than fetal erythrocytes.
B. binds to HbA more avidly than to HbF.
C. increases the affinity of haemoglobin for oxygen.
D. is a phospholipid.
E. is synthesised by the pentose phosphate pathway.

39. Digestive function in a healthy adult involves

A. decreased production of saliva following parasympathetic activity.
B. voluntary oesophageal contractions.
C. release of gastrin from the antral portion of the stomach.
D. delayed gastric emptying after a fatty meal.
E. increased pepsin secretion with vagal stimulation.

40. At puberty

A. the menarche is followed by the growth spurt.
B. early menstrual cycles are frequently anovulatory.
C. the germ cells in the ovary increase in number during this time.
D. the age of menarche is associated with the state of nutrition.
E. the relative size of the uterine body and cervix remains unaltered.

41. The following values fall within the normal range for the adult female bladder:

A. residual urine of 100 ml.
B. voiding volume of 250 ml.
C. bladder capacity of 900 ml.
D. intravesical pressure rise of less than 10 cm H_2O during early filling.
E. maximum urine flow rate of 60 ml per second.

42. The parenchymal cells of the liver

A. can convert fructose to glucose.
B. synthesise urea.
C. conjugate bilirubin.
D. excrete bromsulphthalein.
E. synthesise cholesterol.

43. In the testis

A. maturation from spermatogonia to spermatozoa takes about 29 days.
B. Sertoli cells can mature into spermatids.
C. Leydig cells produce inhibin.
D. luteinising hormone (LH) inhibits the secretion of testosterone.
E. large quantities of fructose are present in seminal fluid.

44. Concerning the vagus nerve:

A. When stimulated, it has little direct effect on the strength of the ventricular contraction.
B. It contains afferent nerve fibres.
C. Stimulation increases the heart rate.
D. It innervates the jejunum.
E. It is involved in the Hering-Breuer reflex.

45. In normal subjects the following increase ventilation:

A. a change in arterial Po_2 from 13.1 KPa (98 mmHg) to 8 KPa (60 mmHg).
B. a change in arterial pH from 7.36 to 7.48.
C. a change in arterial Pco_2 from 5.9 KPa (44 mmHg) to 8 KPa (60 mmHg).
D. administration of doxapram.
E. pregnancy.

46. Calcium in the serum of a healthy adult

A. constitutes 15% of total body calcium.
B. is not involved in the extrinsic system of blood coagulation.
C. concentration is lowered by calcitonin.
D. concentration normally falls after the menopause.
E. is approximately 90% protein-bound.

47. In a healthy, young, nonpregnant woman at rest

A. 80% of the body weight is water.
B. 75% of extracellular fluid is outside the blood vessels.
C. plasma volume is about 5 litres.
D. the pH of the plasma is about 7.25.
E. the plasma osmolality is about 400 mosmol/litre.

48. In the normal adult circulation

A. the pressure in the left ventricle during diastole is twice atmospheric pressure.
B. the aortic blood pressure during diastole is about two-thirds of that during systole.
C. resistance in peripheral blood vessels is inversely proportional to the fourth power of the vessel radius.
D. the arterioles are not subject to sympathetic stimulation except during exercise.
E. increased carotid sinus baroreceptor activity increases the heart rate.

49. Recognised effects of pregnancy include

A. transient impairment of glucose tolerance.
B. a raised glomerular filtration rate.
C. a raised plasma concentration of free tyrosine.
D. a reduced plasma concentration of alkaline phosphatase.
E. an increased secretion of prolactin.

50. The following substances are correctly paired with their site of release:

A. acetylcholine : post-ganglionic parasympathetic nerve endings.
B. noradrenaline : preganglionic sympathetic nerve endings.
C. dopamine : hypothalamus.
D. oxytocin : posterior pituitary.
E. gonadotrophin-releasing hormone : anterior pituitary.

March 2001 Paper 1

1. The anal canal

A. has an upper part which is innervated by the inferior hypogastric plexus.
B. has a lower part which is supplied by the superior rectal artery.
C. drains lymph to the superficial inguinal nodes from its upper part.
D. has its internal sphincter innervated by the inferior rectal nerve.
E. has a superficial part of its external sphincter attached to the coccyx.

2. The pelvic splanchnic nerves

A. are derived from the posterior rami of the sacral spinal nerves.
B. supply afferent fibres.
C. mix with branches of the sympathetic pelvic plexus.
D. supply the ascending colon with motor fibres.
E. supply the uterus with parasympathetic fibres.

3. Concerning histological constituents:

A. The round ligament contains smooth muscle fibres.
B. The bladder epithelium has no mucous glands.
C. The whole of the urethra is lined by squamous epithelium.
D. The sacroiliac joint has a synovial membrane.
E. Skene's glands are present in the clitoris.

4. The following statements about the diaphragm are correct:

A. The greater splanchnic nerves pierce the central tendon.
B. The aortic aperture transmits the thoracic duct.
C. The vena caval aperture transmits the left phrenic nerve.
D. The oesophageal aperture transmits the vagus nerves.
E. Motor fibre supply is by the intercostal nerves.

5. The pudendal nerve

A. arises from the posterior rami of S2, 3 and 4.
B. leaves the pelvis through the lesser sciatic foramen.
C. crosses the ischial spine on the lateral side of the internal pudendal artery.
D. supplies the levator ani.
E. supplies the clitoris.

6. The cervix

A. consists chiefly of smooth muscle.
B. has a supravaginal part which is related anteriorly to the ureter.
C. has a supravaginal part which is covered with peritoneum anteriorly.
D. has pain sensation carried by the pelvic splanchnic nerves.
E. is lined in its vaginal part by keratinised epithelium.

7. In the ovary

A. primordial germ cells are formed.
B. primary oocytes have completed the first mitotic division by birth.
C. the majority of primary oocytes become atretic by puberty.
D. fewer than ten follicles start the process of antrum formation in each ovarian cycle.
E. the second polar body is formed at ovulation.

8. The right ureter lies in close relationship to the

A. bifurcation of the right common iliac artery.
B. infundibulopelvic ligament.
C. uterine artery.
D. inferior mesenteric artery.
E. parietal attachment of the sigmoid mesocolon.

9. The adult female urethra

A. is 7 cm in length.
B. is lined with columnar epithelium in its proximal half.
C. has mucous glands in its distal third.
D. passes through the perineal membrane.
E. is surrounded by smooth muscle in its middle third.

10. The pelvic surface of the sacrum

A. gives origin to the piriformis muscle.
B. gives origin to the levator ani muscle.

C. is broader in the male than in the female.

D. transmits the dorsal rami of sacral nerves.

E. is in contact with the anal canal.

11. Concerning the thigh:

A. Rectus femoris forms the lateral boundary of the femoral triangle.

B. The femoral nerve enters the thigh within the femoral sheath.

C. The ilioinguinal nerve innervates skin over its medial aspect.

D. Both the saphenous nerve and the femoral artery pass through the adductor canal.

E. the lacunar ligament is the medial border of the femoral ring.

12. Concerning the abdominal wall:

A. The umbilicus is located in the territory of the L1 dermatome.

B. The rectus abdominis muscle has attachments to the anterior wall of the rectus sheath.

C. The left and right epigastric arteries anastomose.

D. Distended veins radiating from the umbilicus are indicative of portal hypertension.

E. Langer's lines run vertically over the lower abdomen.

13. Concerning the embryology of the urinary tract:

A. The detrusor has a mesodermal origin.

B. The urogenital sinus is derived from the cloaca.

C. The allantois gives origin to the lateral umbilical ligaments.

D. The ureteric bud arises from the mesonephric duct.

E. The mesonephric duct remnants form the epoophoron in the adult female.

14. In the fetal cardiovascular system

A. the heart arises from endoderm.

B. the heart is formed by fusion of endocardial tubes.

C. cardiac pulsation is present by the 30th day after fertilisation

D. oxygenated blood is transferred from the left atrium through the foramen ovale.

E. the ductus arteriosus closes during the last 4 weeks of pregnancy.

15. Glucagon promotes

A. hepatic gluconeogenesis.

B. glucose uptake by muscle.

C. glycogen synthesis by muscle.
D. breakdown of protein.
E. synthesis of fat.

16. Human insulin

A. is composed of two chains of amino acids.
B. differs from pig insulin by one amino acid.
C. facilitates glucose uptake by red blood cells.
D. increases protein synthesis in the liver.
E. increases triglyceride deposition in adipose tissue.

17. Thyroid hormones

A. increase oxygen consumption in most metabolically active tissues.
B. in the circulation are less than 90% bound to protein.
C. decrease the rate of absorption of carbohydrate from the gut.
D. increase circulating cholesterol concentrations.
E. are essential for skeletal maturation.

18. In congenital adrenal cortical hyperplasia

A. the commonest deficiency is C18 hydroxylase.
B. plasma cortisol concentration is raised.
C. urinary excretion of 17-oxysteroids is elevated.
D. dexamethasone will suppress the urinary excretion of 17-oxysteroids.
E. there are no virilising effects.

19. The corpus luteum of pregnancy produces

A. relaxin.
B. progesterone.
C. 17α-hydroxyprogesterone.
D. human chorionic gonadotrophin.
E. oestradiol.

20. The hypothalamus is the site of synthesis of

A. oxytocin.
B. thyrotrophin-releasing hormone.
C. alpha melanocyte-stimulating hormone.
D. luteinising hormone.
E. gonadotrophin-releasing hormone.

21. Successful lactation is

A. maintained by oestrogens.
B. maintained by progesterone.
C. initiated by a prolactin surge.
D. maintained by human placental lactogen.
E. inhibited by dopamine.

22. Follicle-stimulating hormone

A. binds to a receptor on the cell membrane.
B. promotes the expression of luteinising hormone receptors.
C. is responsible for the degeneration of the corpus luteum.
D. is a steroid hormone.
E. is synthesised in the hypothalamus.

23. Hirsutism in women is characteristically associated with

A. testicular feminisation.
B. Turner syndrome.
C. the polycystic ovary syndrome.
D. arrhenoblastoma.
E. hypopituitarism.

24. Parathyroid hormone

A. decreases the renal excretion of phosphate.
B. increases calcium resorption from bone.
C. depresses pituitary activity.
D. concentrations in blood are raised when the calcium level falls.
E. increases renal tubular reabsorption of calcium.

25. Aldosterone

A. reduces sodium reabsorption in the proximal convoluted tubule.
B. reduces sodium absorption in the descending loop of Henle.
C. increases sodium absorption in the distal convoluted tubule.
D. increases potassium loss from the tubule.
E. increases sodium absorption in the collecting tubule.

26. Human chorionic gonadotrophin

A. is a glycoprotein.
B. secretion peaks at 20 weeks of gestation.
C. has intrinsic anti-thyroid activity.

D.   is synthesised by the corpus luteum of pregnancy.
E.   binds to luteinising hormone receptors.

27. Concerning the renin-angiotensin system:

A.   Renin is secreted by the proximal tubule.
B.   Renin is responsible for the conversion of angiotensin I to angiotensin II.
C.   Angiotensin II is a potent pressor agent.
D.   The pressor effect of angiotensin II is suppressed in normal pregnancy.
E.   Angiotensin II increases the secretion of aldosterone from the adrenal cortex.

28. Ovaries secrete

A.   progesterone.
B.   androstenedione.
C.   testosterone.
D.   17β-oestradiol.
E.   aldosterone.

29. Oestradiol-17β

A.   is synthesised by aromatisation of testosterone.
B.   can be administered orally.
C.   suppresses uterine activity by upregulating the oxytocin receptor.
D.   promotes secondary sexual hair growth in females.
E.   is thrombogenic.

30. Concerning the hypothalamopituitary axis:

A.   Secretion of luteinising hormone is independent of gonadotrophin-releasing hormone.
B.   Gonadotrophin-releasing hormone neurones are absent in Kallman syndrome.
C.   Oestradiol has an acute positive feedback effect on gonadotrophin secretion.
D.   Oestradiol has a chronic negative feedback action on gonadotrophin secretion.
E.   The preovulatory rise in gonadotrophin-releasing hormone secretion is due to an increase in gonadotrophin releasing hormone pulse frequency.

31. The following are RNA-containing viruses:

A. coxsackie.
B. influenza.
C. mumps.
D. herpes simplex.
E. cytomegalovirus.

32. Exotoxins

A. are derived from Gram-negative bacteria.
B. have a specific action.
C. are more toxic than endotoxins.
D. are neutralised by their homologous antitoxin.
E. can be converted to toxoid.

33. *Candida albicans*

A. is a commensal organism in the bowel.
B. is Gram-negative.
C. forms pseudohyphae.
D. is sensitive to gentamicin.
E. reproduces by budding.

34. *Listeria monocytogenes*

A. is a Gram-negative organism.
B. is sensitive to ampicillin.
C. may cause a transplacental infection.
D. is sexually transmitted.
E. can be cultured from a high vaginal swab.

35. Leptospirosis (Weil's disease)

A. produces a positive Wassermann reaction.
B. is associated with jaundice.
C. is transmitted to humans from rats.
D. infection is usually via the skin.
E. is a Rickettsial infection.

36. BCG vaccination of previously uninfected persons

A. produces local erythema within 24 hours.
B. results in regional lymph node enlargement.
C. produces a visible reaction within 3 days.

D. should be given intramuscularly.
E. is ineffective in the newborn.

37. The causative organism of

A. condylomata lata is *Neisseria gonorrhoeae*.
B. chancroid is *Haemophilus ducreyii*.
C. granuloma inguinalae is *Donovania granulomatis*.
D. primary chancre is *Treponema pertenue*.
E. yaws is *Gardnerella vaginalis*.

38. The following organisms are Gram-positive:

A. *Mycobacterium tuberculosis*.
B. *Staphylococcus epidermidis*.
C. *Clostridium perfringens*.
D. *Klebsiella pneumoniae*.
E. *Bacteroides fragilis*.

39. The following drugs should be avoided in renal impairment:

A. cephalothin.
B. cisplatin.
C. norethisterone.
D. dopamine.
E. gentamicin.

40. The following compounds are predominantly progestogens:

A. buserelin.
B. dydrogesterone.
C. norethisterone.
D. 17α-hydroxyprogesterone.
E. androstenedione.

41. The following substances lower the blood glucose concentration:

A. adrenaline.
B. chlorpropamide.
C. chlorothiazide.*
D. metformin.
E. thyroxine.

---

*   This drug has now been discontinued in the UK.

42. The following drugs stimulate myometrial contractility:

A. vasopressin.
B. nifedipine.
C. hydralazine hydrochloride.
D. salbutamol.
E. indomethacin.

43. The following are beta-sympathomimetic effects:

A. constriction of bronchioles.
B. increased heart rate.
C. a decrease in the force of cardiac contraction.
D. constriction of arterioles in the skin.
E. increased glycogenolysis in skeletal muscle.

44. The following statements about anticoagulants are correct:

A. Heparin inhibits the action of thrombin.
B. The action of heparin is antagonised by vitamin K.
C. Heparin increases antithrombin III activity.
D. The effects of coumarin anticoagulants are decreased by metronidazole.
E. Warfarin is greater than 80% protein-bound in plasma.

45. The following stimulate peristalsis in the large bowel:

A. opiates.
B. liquid paraffin.
C. suxamethonium chloride.
D. neostigmine.
E. senna glycoside.

46. The following drugs and sid##fĩ##fĩ##fĩ##fĩsociated:

A. methyldopa: depression.
B. paracetamol: thromboembolism.
C. indomethacin: peptic ulcer.
D. prednisolone: osteoporosis.
E. ritodrine: hypoglycaemia.

47. Co-trimoxazole

A. contains two different drugs.
B. inhibits folic acid synthesis.

C. potentiates the action of warfarin.
D. is bacteriostatic.
E. displaces methotrexate from protein binding sites.

48. One hundred women at high risk of ovarian carcinoma have a pelvic ultrasound scan. The findings after scan and surgery are shown in the table:

Pelvic scan	Ovarian cancer		Total (n)
	Present (n)	Absent (n)	
Abnormal	15	20	35
Normal	5	60	65
Total	20	80	100

A. The sensitivity of the scan is 25% .
B. The specificity of the scan is 75%.
C. The prevalence of ovarian carcinoma is 25%.
D. There are 15 true positive cases.
E. 75% of the patients with ovarian carcinoma had positive scans.

49. Concerning the analysis of clinical trials:

A. The 95% confidence interval indicates the range within which 19 out of 20 values will lie.
B. The P value illustrates how often the result would be expected to occur by chance.
C. The conventional level of statistical significance is set at $P < 0.005$.
D. In a randomised trial, there must be equal numbers of recruits in each arm of the study.
E. A relative risk reduction of 60% is significant irrespective of the value of P.

50. Concerning the ability of a test to predict disease:

A. Sensitivity is the ability to predict those with disease correctly.
B. Sensitivity is the same as positive predictive value.
C. The confidence interval must cross 1 to prove significance.
D. An odds ratio of 1:3 implies a risk of 33%.
E. An odds ratio of 2 indicates a halving of risk.

March 2001
Paper 2

1. Uric acid

A. is formed from the breakdown of purines.
B. serum concentrations are raised during normal pregnancy.
C. serum concentrations are increased during thiazide diuretic therapy.
D. is reabsorbed in the proximal renal tubule.
E. is excreted unchanged in the urine.

2. The level of serum uric acid characteristically

A. falls with starvation.
B. is higher in men than women.
C. rises on taking corticosteroid therapy.
D. falls on treatment with 5 g of aspirin daily.
E. increases in acute leukaemia.

3. Renal sodium retention is favoured by

A. a high glomerular filtration rate.
B. increased secretion of renin.
C. haemoconcentration.
D. expansion of plasma volume.
E. a low renal blood flow.

4. Deficiency of the following substances and diseases are correctly matched:

A. thiamine : pellagra.
B. cyanocobalamin : microcytic anaemia.
C. niacin : beriberi.
D. folates : sprue.
E. ascorbic acid : night blindness.

5. Fetal pulmonary surfactant

A. contains less than 10% lipid.
B. can be detected in amniotic fluid.
C. contains phosphatidylglycerol.
D. is predominantly dipalmitol-phosphatidylcholine.
E. is more than 40% albumin.

6. Potassium

A. is mainly intracellular.
B. plasma levels vary in proportion to intracellular levels.
C. plasma levels are decreased in Addison's disease.
D. plasma levels are increased in diabetic ketoacidosis.
E. deficiency occurs with prolonged vomiting.

7. In the neonate at birth

A. oxygenated haemoglobin is a poorer buffer than deoxygenated haemoglobin.
B. more than 50% of the circulating haemoglobin is haemoglobin F.
C. oxygen dissociation from haemoglobin is promoted by acidosis.
D. the total haemoglobin concentration is generally above 15 g/dl.
E. red blood cell 2,3-diphosphoglyceric acid is absent.

8. DNA

A. contains no cytosine.
B. has a backbone of ribose.
C. is usually single stranded in mammalian cells.
D. is cleaved by restriction enzymes.
E. is irreversibly damaged in vitro by heating to 75°C.

9. Glycogen

A. is a polymer of glucose residues.
B. is predominantly found in cytoplasm.
C. is mainly stored in the liver.
D. is cleaved by phosphorylase.
E. breakdown is inhibited by adrenaline.

10. Biochemical abnormalities associated with diabetes mellitus include

A.   increased breakdown of protein.
B.   decreased plasma levels of free fatty acids.
C.   increased serum cholesterol concentrations.
D.   decreased glycosylation of haemoglobin.
E.   a decrease in the plasma concentration of low density lipoproteins.

11. Concerning carbohydrates:

A.   Sucrose is a disaccharide of glucose and fructose.
B.   Cereal grains contain less than 40% starch.
C.   Cellulose is a fructose polysaccharide.
D.   A normal diet contains less than 60 g of carbohydrate daily.
E.   Dietary carbohydrate is oxidised in the body to carbon dioxide and water.

12. Muscle glycogen

A.   metabolism cannot yield free glucose.
B.   metabolism is independent of the enzyme phosphorylase.
C.   metabolism only generates ATP under aerobic conditions.
D.   is entirely intracellular.
E.   is released into the circulation in response to glucocorticoids.

13. The following result in metabolic acidosis:

A.   ketoacidosis.
B.   muscular exercise.
C.   renal failure.
D.   hypoxia.
E.   acute respiratory failure.

14. L-glucose is

A.   a pentose.
B.   an aldose.
C.   a ketose.
D.   a mirror image of D-glucose.
E.   identical in biological activity to D-glucose.

15. Glucose

A.   is predominantly absorbed in the terminal ileum.
B.   stimulates the secretion of glucagon.

C. can be synthesised from pyruvate.
D. is a disaccharide.
E. is the only metabolic substrate for cardiac muscle.

16. Concerning radiation physics:

A. An electron has a greater mass than a proton.
B. A positron has the same charge as an electron.
C. A proton has a positive charge.
D. A neutron has almost the same mass as a proton.
E. The hydrogen nucleus is a neutron.

17. Messenger RNA (mRNA)

A. synthesis is catalysed by RNA polymerase II.
B. is an exact copy of sense DNA.
C. contains exons.
D. is measured by Western analysis.
E. translation occurs in the nucleus.

18. Concerning the genetic control of protein synthesis:

A. Mature messenger RNA contains introns.
B. A codon has 3-base sequences.
C. Each amino acid has a single codon.
D. Transfer RNA has anticodon recognition sites.
E. Each transfer RNA carries a specific amino acid.

19. In an X-linked pedigree

A. none of the sons of an affected father will be affected.
B. half of the daughters of an affected male will not carry the gene.
C. half of the sons of carrier females will be affected.
D. females are never affected.
E. all of the daughters of a carrier female will themselves be carriers.

20. The following genes and chromosomes are correctly paired:

A. HLA : chromosome 6.
B. clotting factor VIII : X chromosome.
C. glucose-6-phosphate dehydrogenase : X chromosome.
D. testis determining factor : X chromosome.
E. Xg blood group : chromosome 1.

21. In the human, a haploid number of chromosomes is found in

A. red blood cells.
B. blastocysts.
C. primary oocytes.
D. the first polar body.
E. spermatozoa.

22. Plasma cells

A. are increased in myeloma.
B. are characteristic of acute infection.
C. are phagocytic.
D. synthesise irmnunoglobulins.
E. are derived from B lymphocytes.

23. The following are recognised functions of T lymphocytes:

A. antibody production.
B. cell mediated immunity.
C. immune regulation.
D. phagocytosis.
E. cytokine production.

24. Tissue macrophages

A. are found in the placental villous stroma.
B. express HLA class I but not HLA class II surface antigens.
C. have a role in protection against intracellular pathogens.
D. are phagocytic.
E. are derived from circulating plasma cells.

25. Osteoporosis is associated with

A. an increase in uncalcified bone matrix.
B. prolonged oestrogen therapy.
C. long term heparin treatment.
D. bone fractures.
E. irregularity of epiphyseal plates.

26. The following are X-linked disorders:

A. myotonic dystrophy
B. Duchenne muscular dystrophy
C. haemophilia A

D. Huntington's disease
E. fragile X syndrome

27. A metaplastic process is involved in the histogenesis of the following tumours:

A. squamous cell carcinoma of the vulva.
B. squamous cell carcinoma of the bronchus.
C. scirrhous carcinoma of the breast.
D. adenocarcinoma of the cervix.
E. adenocarcinoma of the ovary.

28. Amyloid

A. is predominantly intracellular.
B. contains fibrils.
C. is enzymatic.
D. can be found in nerve tissue.
E. deposits occur with chronic sepsis.

29. The following tumours are correctly paired with likely causative agents:

A. angiocarcinoma of the liver : vinyl chloride.
B. carcinoma of the colon : dietary fibre.
C. hepatoma : aflatoxins.
D. carcinoma of the bronchus : coal dust.
E. carcinoma of the bladder : beta naphthylamine.

30. Tetany may occur as a complication of

A. osteoporosis.
B. hypercapnia.
C. respiratory acidosis.
D. peripheral neuropathy.
E. untreated hyperparathyroidism.

31. Stored blood which is to be used for transfusion

A. is kept at −4°C.
B. must be used within 1 week.
C. is tested for complement content before transfusion.
D. may be used for platelet replacement.
E. contains an acid anticoagulant.

32. In uncomplicated homozygous beta thalassaemia there is

A. hypochromasia.
B. a reduction in haemoglobin A_2.
C. an increase in haemoglobin F.
D. megaloblastic erythropoiesis.
E. red cell sickling.

33. Neutrophil polymorphs at the site of inflammation are capable of the following:

A. phagocytosis.
B. production of oxygen free radicals.
C. replication.
D. fusion to form giant cells.
E. antibody production.

34. The following are consequences of pulmonary embolism:

A. pulmonary infarction.
B. fibrinous pleurisy.
C. right ventricular hypertrophy.
D. sudden death.
E. haemoptysis.

35. Apoptosis

A. causes necrotic cell death.
B. is involved in embryonic remodelling.
C. releases pro-inflammatory mediators.
D. is characterised by condensation of nuclear chromatin.
E. is associated with endonuclease activity.

36. Concerning cells:

A. Glycosylation takes place in the smooth endoplasmic reticulum.
B. Low density lipoproteins attach to cell membrane receptors.
C. Glycoproteins are present on the cytosol surface of the plasma membrane.
D. Centrioles are composed of tubulin.
E. Nuclear heterochromatin is genetically inactive.

37. Concerning oxygenation of fetal blood:

A. The fetal-maternal Pco_2 gradient facilitates maternal–fetal oxygen transfer.

B. fetal haemoglobin is less influenced by 2,3-diphosphoglyceric acid concentration than adult haeroglobin.
C. The fetal blood oxygen dissociation curve lies to the right of the maternal curve.
D. The uptake of oxygen decreases fetal red cell buffering capacity.
E. Uptake of oxygen by fetal blood is associated with a shift of chloride into fetal red cells.

38. The Leydig cells of the testis

A. secrete seminal fluid.
B. are stimulated by luteinising hormone.
C. are active in intrauterine life.
D. secrete fructose.
E. produce androstenedione.

39. In the nonpregnant woman during the cardiac cycle:

A. atrial contraction occurs in the early stages of ventricular filling.
B. adrenergic stimulation increases the heart rate.
C. the first heart sound is caused by closure of the aortic valves.
D. stroke volume at rest is 200 ml.
E. the peak pressure in the pulmonary arterial system is less than one-tenth of that in the systemic circulation.

40. The blood concentrations of the following are lowered in pregnancy:

A. bicarbonate.
B. transferrin.
C. sodium.
D. albumin.
E. fibrinogen.

41. Plasminogen is

A. alpha globulin.
B. activated by α_2-macroglobulin.
C. inhibited by streptokinase.
D. formed from plasmin.
E. released from plasma cells.

42. The conjugation of bilirubin

A. takes place in hepatocytes.

B.   is catalysed by UDP glucuronyl transferase.
C.   is inhibited by phenobarbitone.
D.   renders it water soluble.
E.   is impaired in acute biliary obstruction.

43. Angiotensin II

A.   is a vasoconstrictor.
B.   reduces aldosterone production.
C.   is mainly found in the lungs.
D.   is a decapeptide.
E.   is produced when the extracellular fluid volume is reduced.

44. The following factors increase ventilation in normal women:

A.   a rise in P_{CO_2} from 5.3 KPa to 8.0 KPa (40–50 mmHg).
B.   a fall in P_{O_2} from 13.1 KPa to 11.7 KPa (98–88 mmHg).
C.   pregnancy.
D.   a fall in pH from 7.4 to 7.3.
E.   taking a combined oral contraceptive pill.

45. The stroke volume of the left ventricle

A.   is equal to the blood volume in the ventricle at the end of diastole.
B.   may be increased without increasing the end diastolic volume of the ventricle.
C.   is directly related to the duration of the previous diastolic pause.
D.   is consistently greater than that of the right ventricle.
E.   is 20–30 ml in a resting man of average size in the supine position

46. In normal pregnancy, uterine blood flow

A.   is about 50 ml/minute at term.
B.   within the choriodecidual space is maintained throughout the cardiac cycle.
C.   is reduced by prostacyclin.
D.   is increased during uterine contractions.
E.   represents about 10% of the cardiac output by the end of the first trimester.

47. The following increase during normal pregnancy

A.   the basal metabolic rate.
B.   serum cholesterol concentration.
C.   fasting blood glucose concentration.

D.   serum sodium concentration.
E.   serum fibrinogen concentration.

48.   Physiological changes associated with pregnancy include

A.   a rise in erythrocyte sedimentation rate.
B.   a rise in total body haemoglobin.
C.   a fall in plasma fibrinogen concentration.
D.   an increase in the total number of leucocytes.
E.   an increase in blood urea concentration within the first trimester.

49.   Concerning human parturition:

A.   The number of oxytocin receptors in the myometrium increases before the onset of labour.
B.   In the primigravida cervical dilatation usually precedes cervical effacement.
C.   The plasma oxytocin concentration increases at the onset of labour.
D.   Oxytocin stimulates the synthesis of prostaglandins within the uterus.
E.   Contraction of the maternal abdominal muscles is essential for spontaneous vaginal delivery.

50.   In normal pregnancy

A.   trophoblast cells initially invade uterine spiral arterioles at 16–18 weeks of gestation.
B.   villous cytotrophoblast forms a layer beneath the syncytiotrophoblast in early pregnancy.
C.   the syncytiotrophoblast is the only cellular layer between maternal and fetal blood.
D.   syncytial knots in the placenta are composed of aggregates of cytotrophoblast.
E.   trophoblast cells invade the myometrium.

September 2001 Paper 1

1. The vagina

A. is lined by squamous epithelium.
B. is supplied in part by the uterine artery.
C. is covered with peritoneum in its upper anterior aspect.
D. has venous drainage to the external iliac vein.
E. is supplied in part by the pudendal nerve.

2. The following muscles are inserted into the perineal body:

A. bulbospongiosus.
B. ischiocavernosus.
C. obturator internus.
D. external anal sphincter.
E. superficial transverse perineal.

3. In the abdominal wall

A. the rectus abdominis muscle is attached to the crest of the pubis.
B. the posterior border of the external oblique muscle ends in the linea semilunaris.
C. the aponeurosis of the external oblique muscle takes part in the formation of the conjoint tendon.
D. the inferior epigastric artery is a branch of the internal iliac artery.
E. the conjoint tendon blends medially with the anterior layer of the rectus sheath.

4. In the pituitary gland

A. the anterior lobe is smaller than the posterior lobe.
B. the posterior lobe is ectodermal in origin.
C. the acidophil cells produce oxytocin.
D. the basophil cells produce growth hormone.
E. the blood supply is derived from the internal carotid artery.

5.   The pineal gland

A.   is situated at the anterior end of the third ventricle.
B.   is innervated by the parasympathetic nervous system.
C.   produces melatonin.
D.   may be calcified in the adult.
E.   is most active during daylight.

6.   The pelvic splanchnic nerves

A.   are derived from the posterior rami of the sacral spinal nerves.
B.   supply afferent fibres.
C.   intermingle with branches of the sympathetic pelvic plexus.
D.   supply the ascending colon with motor fibres.
E.   supply the uterus with parasympathetic fibres.

7.   The parasympathic nervous system supplies

A.   dilator fibres to the bronchioles.
B.   constrictor fibres to the small intestine.
C.   inhibitory fibres to the myocardium.
D.   dilator fibres to the sphincter pupillae.
E.   constrictor fibres to the detrusor muscle.

8.   The ovary

A.   is attached to the anterior surface of the broad ligament.
B.   lies on the genitofemoral nerve.
C.   lies in the angle between the ureter and the external iliac vessels.
D.   has visceral afferent fibres from the pelvic splanchnic nerves.
E.   has lymphatic drainage to the superficial inguinal lymph nodes.

9.   The ureter

A.   is supplied in part by the ovarian artery.
B.   lies lateral to the transverse processes of the lumbar vertebrae.
C.   passes above the genitofemoral nerve.
D.   is lined by simple columnar epithelium.
E.   passes beneath the uterine artery.

10. In the normal human pelvis

A.   the promontory of the sacrum is the upper anterior border of the
     first sacral vertebra.
B.   the anterior surface of the sacrum has five paired foramina.

C. the joint between the two pubic bones is a synovial joint.
D. the acetabular fossa is wholly formed from parts of the pubic and ischial bones.
E. the transverse diameter of the brim is greater than the antero-posterior diameter.

11. The femoral ring

A. has the pectineal ligament lying medial to it.
B. is in contact with the femoral artery.
C. has the lacunar ligament lying anterior to it.
D. contains a lymph node that drains the clitoris.
E. has the femoral sheath lying anterior, posterior and medial to it.

12. Concerning the uterus:

A. It is formed from the mesonephric ducts.
B. It has a lympatic drainage in part to the inguinal glands.
C. The uterine artery passes below the ureter.
D. The uterine veins communicate with the vesical plexus of veins.
E. Pain sensation from the body of the uterus is carried by the pelvic splanchnic nerves.

13. The mesoderm gives rise to

A. striated muscle.
B. blood.
C. peritoneum.
D. transitional epithelium of the bladder.
E. ovarian stroma.

14. Concerning embryological development:

A. The amnion has an endodermal origin.
B. Uterine epithelium is developed from the paramesonephric duct.
C. The ducts of Bartholin's glands open above the hymen.
D. The round ligament of the uterus is derived from the gubernaculum.
E. The adrenal cortex is derived from neural crest cells.

15. Concerning insulin:

A. The half-life of endogenous insulin in the circulation is 30 minutes.
B. The kidney is a major site of insulin degradation.
C. It facilitates glucose uptake by the brain.

D. Fasting concentrations are lower in pregnant women at term than they are in nonpregnant women.
E. It is formed when C-peptide is separated from proinsulin.

16. Iodine

A. requirements are unchanged by pregnancy.
B. uptake by the thyroid gland is increased by thyroid stimulating hormone.
C. is excreted by the kidney.
D. is bound to tyrosine in the thyroid gland.
E. may inhibit thyroxine synthesis.

17. Concerning thyroid function:

A. Oestrogen increases the production of thyroxine-binding globulin.
B. More than 98% of circulating thyroxine is bound to thyroxine-binding globulin.
C. Thyrotrophin-releasing hormone is a decapeptide.
D. Thyroid-stimulating hormone levels are increased in primary hypothyroidism.
E. Thyroid-stimulating hormone is a glycoprotein.

18. The interstitial (Leydig) cells of the testis

A. secrete seminal fluid.
B. are stimulated by luteinising hormone.
C. secrete androgen binding protein.
D. secrete fructose.
E. produce testosterone.

19. During the normal ovarian cycle

A. the principle oestrogen secreted is 17β-oestradiol.
B. the most potent oestrogen is oestriol.
C. oestrogen production is maximal by about the eighth day of the cycle.
D. oestrogens decrease the secretion of follicle-stimulating hormone.
E. oestrogens are synthesised primarily by the ovarian stroma.

20. Testosterone

A. is produced only in the gonads.
B. is mainly excreted unchanged in the urine.

C. stimulates secretion of luteinising hormone.
D. circulates in plasma mainly in the free form.
E. stimulates growth of the prostate gland.

21. Progesterone

A. is synthesised by trophoblast.
B. increases myometrial activity.
C. is predominantly excreted in the urine as pregnanetriol.
D. binds to cortisol-binding globulin in the circulation.
E. is synthesised from cholesterol.

22. During human lactation

A. oxytocin increases mammary duct pressure.
B. oestrogens promote the milk-producing effects of prolactin on the breast.
C. human placental lactogen is essential for milk synthesis.
D. prolactin stimulates gonadotrophin release.
E. suckling enhances prolactin release.

23. The following statements concerning the formation of hormones are correct:

A. ACTH is derived from pro-opiomelanocortin.
B. Oestrogens are derived from androgens.
C. Prolactin is derived from dopamine.
D. Melatonin is derived from serotonin.
E. Angiotensin II is derived from rennin.

24. Pituitary gonadotrophin

A. release is dependent on hypothalamic function.
B. secretion increases during pregnancy.
C. blood levels are raised during lactational amenorrhoea.
D. release in the puerperium is enhanced by bromocriptine.
E. release is inhibited by oxytocin.

25. Adrenaline (epinephrine)

A. stimulates myometrial contractions.
B. exerts its action by alpha receptors only.
C. constricts the pupils.
D. causes glycogenolysis.
E. inhibits the mobilisation of free fatty acids.

26. Prolactin

A. release is stimulated by thyrotrophin-releasing hormone.
B. plasma levels are raised in the first trimester of pregnancy.
C. release is increased by suckling.
D. may be produced by the decidua.
E. release is inhibited by metoclopramide.

27. Growth hormone

A. is a protein.
B. has a molecular weight of 2000 Daltons.
C. secretion is stimulated by hyperglycaemia.
D. has growth-promoting effects mediated through insulin-like growth factors.
E. is synthesised in the hypothalamus.

28. Arginine vasopressin

A. reduces glomerular filtration rate.
B. controls water loss in the proximal renal tubule.
C. is synthesised by the posterior pituitary gland.
D. is released in response to a rise in plasma osmolality.
E. is released in response to a fall in circulating plasma volume.

29. Parathyroid hormone

A. increases bone resorption.
B. concentrations are increased in pregnancy.
C. reduces phosphate excretion in urine.
D. increases the formation of 1,25-dihydroxycholecalciferol.
E. stimulates osteoblasts.

30. The following hormones bind to receptors on the cell membrane:

A. corticosterone.
B. adrenaline.
C. luteinising hormone.
D. oestradiol.
E. gonadotrophin-releasing hormone.

31. Steroid hormones

A. all contain 20 carbon atoms.
B. can be produced by structures of urogenital ridge origin.

C.   are mostly activated in the liver.
D.   are predominantly excreted unchanged in the urine.
E.   mainly circulate unbound to carrier proteins.

32. Bacteroides

A.   are motile.
B.   do not produce spores.
C.   grow in aerobic culture.
D.   are synergistic coli forms.
E.   are characteristically resistant to penicillin.

33. In septic shock

A.   the causative organisms are invariably Gram-negative
B.   death is characterised by leucocytosis.
C.   endotoxins are predominantly lipopolysaccharides.
D.   antibiotic treatment may aggravate hypotension.
E.   there may be associated disseminated intravascular coagulation.

34. Toxic shock syndrome in women

A.   is associated with the use of tampons.
B.   is due to a toxogenic strain of streptococcus.
C.   has induction of nitric oxide as a pathogenic feature.
D.   is infrequently reported outside North America.
E.   is confined to sexually active women.

35. Chlamydia organisms

A.   are motile.
B.   are intracellular.
C.   infect squamous cells.
D.   are found in birds.
E.   cause trachoma.

36. Mycobacteria

A.   are non-sporing.
B.   are all acid-fast in their staining reaction.
C.   are facultative anaerobes.
D.   are responsible for leprosy.
E.   are all pathogenic in humans

37. Concerning viral infections:

A. Cytomegalovirus is of the herpes group.
B. Herpes simplex virus may remain dormant in epithelial cells of the lower genital tract.
C. Facial herpes simplex lesions are activated by sunlight.
D. Coxsackie B virus does not cross the placenta.
E. Hepatitis B virus may be sexually transmitted.

38. Concerning *Neisseria*:

A. *N. meningitidis* can be a nasopharyngeal commensal.
B. *N. gonorrhoeae* will grow in anaerobic conditions.
C. *N. gonorrhoeae* culture is inhibited at low temperatures.
D. *N. gonorrhoeae* is identified within the cytoplasm of polymorphs.
E. *N. gonorrhoeae* infection can cause an arthropathy.

39. The following drugs are potassium-sparing diuretics:

A. amiloride hydrochloride.
B. triamterene.
C. spironolactone.
D. chlorothiazide.*
E. frusemide.**

40. The following drugs may cause enlargement of the fetal thyroid gland:

A. methyldopa.
B. thyroxine.
C. carbimazole.
D. propranolol.
E. propylthiouracil.

41. The following statements describe the action of drugs on the myometrium:

A. Ergometrine stimulates sympathetic alpha receptors.
B. Indomethacin inhibits contractions by blocking prostaglandin receptors.
C. Prostaglandin E_1 is a stimulant of isolated uterine tissue *in vitro*.
D. Oxytocin requires ionised calcium as a cofactor.
E. Magnesium sulphate is a myometrial stimulant.

---

*   This drug has now been discontinued in the UK.
** Registered non-proprietary name is furosemide; BNF 48, September 2004.

42. The following are cytotoxic alkylating agents:

A. cyclophosphamide.
B. mercaptopurine.
C. chlorambucil.
D. fluorouracil.
E. methotrexate.

43. Treatment with morphine

A. causes respiratory depression.
B. increases gastric motility.
C. causes side effects, all of which may be reversed.
D. increases the secretion of anti-diuretic hormone.
E. causes pupillary dilatation.

44. The following substances increase the serum uric acid concentration:

A. colchicine.
B. chlorothiazide.*
C. allopurinol.
D. probenecid.
E. phenylbutazone.**

45. The following statements are true:

A. Suxamethonium is a non-depolarising muscle relaxant.
B. Hexamethonium is a ganglion blocker.
C. Tubocurarine is reversed by neostigmine.
D. Streptomycin is absorbed from the gastrointestinal tract.
E. Thiopentone can be given intramuscularly.

46. The following are features of ergometrine maleate:

A. it is inactive when administered orally.
B. the onset of action after intravenous injection occurs in approximately 5 minutes.
C. transient hypertension may occur after its administration.
D. parenteral administration may result in vomiting.
E. its use is contraindicated in patients with migraine.

---

* Discontinued in the UK, September 2002.
** This drug has now been discontinued in the UK.

47. A normal distribution of values

A. is symmetrical about the mode.
B. has a median which is greater than the mean.
C. has 75% of its values below the upper quartile.
D. may contain negative values.
E. allows calculation of the standard deviation.

48. The following statistical statements are correct:

A. In the normal distribution, the value of the mode is 1.73 x that of the median.
B. In a distribution skewed to the right, the mean lies to the left of the median.
C. In the series: 2; 7; 5; 2; 3; 2; 5; 8, the mode is 2.
D. Student's *t*-test is designed to correct for skew distribution.
E. The Chi-squared test may be used when data are not normally distributed.

49. In a clinical trial, randomised allocation of patients to treatment groups

A. eliminates the investigator's bias.
B. reduces the placebo effect.
C. usually controls for known confounding variables.
D. usually controls for unknown confounding variables.
E. is best achieved by alternate allocation of subjects.

50. In randomised double-blind trial comparing a new drug with a placebo,

A. the patients will be taking either of two active drugs.
B. patients can choose their method of treatment.
C. doctors prescribing treatment decide which patients take the new drug.
D. a large trial is more likely to give a statistically significant result than a small trial.
E. exactly 50% of the patients will take the new drug.

September 2001 Paper 2

1. Ketone bodies

A. can be utilised by the fetal brain.
B. include aceto-acetate.
C. are water soluble.
D. are synthesised in skeletal muscle.
E. can be utilised during starvation.

2. Intracellular fluid differs from extracellular fluid in that

A. it forms the larger proportion of total body water.
B. its volume can be more readily measured.
C. it has a higher concentration of potassium.
D. its volume is more directly regulated by the kidneys.
E. it has a lower concentration of sodium.

3. The oxidation of pyruvate to carbon dioxide

A. occurs exclusively in mitochondria.
B. can occur under anaerobic conditions.
C. involves intermediates that are also involved in amino acid catabolism.
D. is regulated by the concentration of acetyl coenzyme A in the cell.
E. is impaired in thiamine deficiency states.

4. Creatinine

A. is filtered out by the glomerulus.
B. is reabsorbed significantly by the proximal tubules.
C. plasma concentration increases after protein ingestion.
D. has a plasma clearance rate equivalent to renal plasma flow.
E. plasma concentration increases during the first trimester of pregnancy.

5. ABO antigens are

A. glycoproteins.
B. found only on erythrocytes.
C. major histocompatibility antigens.
D. not immunogenic during pregnancy.
E. located on membranes.

6. Haemoglobin

A. has four porphyrin rings.
B. can carry four molecules of oxygen.
C. binds carbon monoxide more readily than oxygen.
D. is synthesised in mature erythrocytes.
E. contains two beta chains.

7. Iron

A. is altered to the ferric state after absorption.
B. is transported by apoferritin.
C. is readily excreted by the kidney.
D. retention in the body is enhanced by chelating agents.
E. requirement during normal pregnancy is approximately 1 mg per day.

8. Cholecalciferol (vitamin D)

A. promotes the absorption of calcium from the gut.
B. is 25-hydroxylated in the liver.
C. is synthesised in the skin.
D. is 1-hydroxylated in the kidney.
E. is most active in the 1,25-dihydroxyl form.

9. Excess

A. vitamin C causes haemorrhage.
B. vitamin D causes renal failure.
C. vitamin K causes thrombosis.
D. vitamin E causes azoospermia.
E. vitamin A causes headache.

10. Folic acid

A. requires gastric intrinsic factor for its absorption.
B. daily requirement is about 40 mg.
C. is found in higher concentration in fetal blood than in maternal blood.

D.   deficiency leads to microcytic anaemia.
E.   is fat soluble.

11. The conjugation of bilirubin

A.   takes place in hepatocytes.
B.   is catalysed by UDP glucuronyl transferase.
C.   is inhibited by phenobarbitone.
D.   renders it water soluble.
E.   is impaired in acute biliary obstruction.

12. Messenger ribonucleic acid (mRNA)

A.   is a double-stranded polymer.
B.   is transcribed from DNA in the nucleus.
C.   is not present in reticulocytes.
D.   contains thymine.
E.   is not present in oocytes.

13. Concerning glycolysis:

A.   it is the mobilisation of stored glucose units.
B.   most of the reactions occur in the mitochondria.
C.   two molecules of ATP (adenosine triphosphate) are consumed per molecule of glucose.
D.   there is a net gain of two ATP molecules from the conversion of a glucose molecule to two pyruvate molecules.
E.   the glucose to pyruvate pathway is present in all tissues.

14. The following substances are normally synthesised in the liver:

A.   glucagon.
B.   vitamin A.
C.   cholesterol.
D.   immunoglobulins.
E.   prothrombin.

15. Hyperkalaemia is a characteristic finding in

A.   primary aldosteronism.
B.   treatment with spironolactone.
C.   hyperparathyroidism.
D.   adrenocorticotrophic hormone-secreting tumours of the bronchus.
E.   renal failure.

16. The natural decay of radioactive isotopes results in the emission of

A. alpha particles.
B. gamma rays.
C. neutron rays.
D. proton beams.
E. beta particles.

17. In radiotherapy

A. one Gray is equivalent to one joule per kilogram.
B. the skin usually receives a greater dose of radiation than the underlying tissues.
C. the major effect of radiation energy is to damage the cytoplasm of the cell.
D. cells in tissues which are hypoxic are more vulnerable to radiation.
E. radiation-induced changes in tissues may take 6 weeks to develop.

18. A woman who has a rhesus (Rh) genotype of Cde/CDe

A. could develop anti-C antibodies.
B. could safely be transfused with D positive blood.
C. may develop anti-E antibodies.
D. should receive anti-D immunoglobulin after giving birth to a Rh (D) positive infant.
E. is Rh negative.

19. When a man has haemophilia

A. 50% of his daughters would not expect to be carriers.
B. 25% of his sons would be expected to be affected.
C. good medical control of his blood deficiency reduces the risk of the condition in his children.
D. his newborn child is likely to require an urgent blood transfusion.
E. his sister has a 50% probability of being a carrier.

20. In the neonate, the appearance of the external genitalia may not correspond with the genotype in the presence of

A. adrenogenital syndrome.
B. testicular feminisation syndrome.
C. renal agenesis (Potter syndrome).
D. trisomy 21.
E. severe hypospadias.

21. Concerning inheritable diseases:

A. Huntingdon's chorea is transmitted by a dominant gene.
B. phenylketonuria is transmitted by a recessive gene.
C. haemophilia is an autosomal dominant condition.
D. von Willebrand's disease is a sex-linked condition.
E. cystic fibrosis is transmitted by an X-linked recessive gene.

22. Concerning the genetic control of protein synthesis:

A. Mature mRNA contains introns.
B. A codon has 3-base sequences.
C. Each amino acid has a single codon.
D. Transfer RNA (tRNA) has anticodon recognition sites.
E. Each tRNA carries a specific amino acid.

23. The human major histocompatibility complex (MHC) genes

A. map to chromosome 11.
B. are composed of human leucocyte antigen (HLA) genes.
C. are the most polymorphic in the human genome.
D. will be identical in dizygotic twins.
E. code for blood group antigens.

24. The following cells are correctly paired with their products:

A. endothelial cell : factor VIII-related antigen.
B. plasma cell : IgG.
C. salivary gland epithelial cell : amylase.
D. mast cell : IgA.
E. decidual stromal cell : prolactin.

25. Immunodeficiency states may be associated with:

A. viral infection of T lymphocytes.
B. B cell lymphomata.
C. glucocorticoid administration.
D. haemolytic disease of the newborn.
E. Hodgkin's lymphoma.

26. The following are autosomal recessive diseases:

A. neurofibromatosis.
B. cystic fibrosis.
C. phenylketonuria.

D.   polyposis coli.
E.   sickle cell anaemia.

27. The following cells may be phagocytic:

A.   neutrophils.
B.   Kupffer cells.
C.   monocytes.
D.   Hoffbauer cells.
E.   plasma cells.

28. The following tumours produce characteristic blood markers:

A.   clear cell carcinoma.
B.   choriocarcinoma.
C.   osteogenic sarcoma.
D.   yolk sac tumour.
E.   transitional cell tumour.

29. The following pairs indicate correct pathological association:

A.   Epstein-Barr virus : Burkitt's lymphoma.
B.   Peutz-Jeghers syndrome : intestinal carcinoma.
C.   wood dust : pleural mesothelioma.
D.   progestogens : endometrial carcinoma.
E.   aniline dyes : bladder carcinoma.

30. Growth of the following tumours is hormone-dependent:

A.   squamous cell carcinoma of the cervix.
B.   breast adenocarcinoma.
C.   uterine leiomyoma.
D.   prostatic adenocarcinoma.
E.   testicular carcinoma.

31. Rickets is characterised by the following:

A.   mineralisation of the periosteum.
B.   deposition of uncalcified osteoid.
C.   abnormal osteoblastic activity.
D.   increased capillary fragility.
E.   overgrowth of cartilage.

32. The following tissues are capable of cellular regeneration:

A. spinal cord.
B. liver.
C. epidermis.
D. myocardium.
E. bone marrow.

33. Oxygen

A. binds to trivalent iron in the haem molecule.
B. is carried as four molecules per molecule of haemoglobin.
C. -haemoglobin dissociation is linear.
D. uptake reduces red cell buffering capacity.
E. is released from haemoglobin when the concentration of 2,3-diphosphoglyceric acid is decreased.

34. Intracellular concentration of free calcium

A. is greater than that of extracellular free calcium.
B. may be influenced by voltage-gated membrane channels.
C. may be influenced by the activity of inositol triphosphate.
D. binds to calmodulin.
E. inactivates troponin C.

35. Displacement of oxyhaemoglobin dissociation to the right

A. means a greater avidity of haemoglobin for oxygen.
B. occurs immediately on ascent to high altitude.
C. occurs with a rise in temperature.
D. occurs with a fall in pH.
E. occurs with a fall in Pco_2.

36. Platelets

A. are approximately 50 micrometers in diameter.
B. contain myosin.
C. release a growth factor.
D. are formed from myeloblasts.
E. are prevented from aggregating by thromboxane A_2.

37. In uncomplicated homozygous beta thalassaemia there is

A. hypochromasia.
B. a reduction in haemoglobin A_2.

C. an increase in haemoglobin F.
D. no depletion of iron stores.
E. the presence of megaloblasts in bone marrow.

38. In the nephron, sodium

A. is mainly reabsorbed in the proximal convoluted tubule.
B. reabsorption increases in normal pregnancy.
C. may be reabsorbed in exchange for hydrogen ions.
D. reabsorption is increased by spironolactone.
E. reabsorption is increased by atrial natriuretic peptide.

39. Bile

A. production is inhibited after vagal stimulation.
B. is concentrated under the influence of secretin.
C. has a pH of 5.5.
D. is expelled from the gall bladder under the influence of cholecystokinin.
E. normally contains high concentrations of free cholesterol.

40. Bradykinin

A. increases capillary permeability.
B. is a small polypeptide.
C. is formed by the action of kallikrein.
D. is predominantly inactivated in the liver.
E. is metabolised to kininogen.

41. 'Physiological' jaundice of the newborn

A. is present on the first day of life.
B. is due to ABO incompatibility.
C. is associated with a raised serum concentration of glutamic pyruvic transaminase.
D. may be due to relative glucuronyl transferase deficiency.
E. is associated with a raised level of unconjugated bilirubin.

42. The stimulation of adrenergic alpha receptors

A. does not occur with noradrenaline.
B. in the blood vessels of the skin leads to vasoconstriction.
C. in the gastrointestinal sphincter muscles leads to relaxation.
D. in the iris leads to constriction of the pupil.
E. in the blood vessels of the kidney leads to vasodilatation.

43. In a normal man breathing quietly at rest, the partial pressure of

A. carbon dioxide in alveolar air is about three times greater than in room air.
B. nitrogen is greater in expired air than in inspired air.
C. water vapour in alveolar air is less than in room air.
D. carbon dioxide in the blood of the pulmonary arteries is greater than in alveolar air.
E. oxygen is less in the pulmonary veins than in alveolar air.

44. Total body water

A. forms a smaller proportion of body water in fat than thin persons.
B. can be measured by a deuterium oxide dilution technique.
C. normally comprises 45–65% of body weight.
D. is a smaller proportion of body weight in men than in women.
E. is predominantly intracellular.

45. Concerning blood pressure regulation:

A. Adrenaline acts primarily upon the vasomotor centre.
B. Prostacyclin lowers blood pressure.
C. Angiotensinogen is inactive without modification.
D. Bradykinin increases blood pressure.
E. Serotonin is vasodilatory.

46. During normal pregnancy

A. arterial Pco_2 decreases.
B. the blood hydrogen ion concentration decreases.
C. plasma bicarbonate concentrations decrease.
D. urine pH falls.
E. lactic acid production is increased.

47. Concerning the fetal cardiovascular system:

A. More than 80% of the cardiac output flows through the placenta.
B. Oxygen saturation in the carotid and renal arteries is the same.
C. Umbilical venous blood has a lower Po_2 than renal arterial blood.
D. Blood from the inferior vena cava passes directly into the left ventricle.
E. The pulmonary circulation has a high resistance.

48. The partial pressure of carbon dioxide in arterial blood may be raised in

A. residence at high altitude.
B. gross obesity.
C. acidaemia due to renal failure.
D. hyperventilation.
E. pregnancy.

49. In the lungs of a healthy male adult at rest

A. alveolar air contains 40% nitrogen.
B. about 2 litres of air are in the alveoli at the end of a quiet expiration.
C. about 150 ml of inspired air in each breath do not reach the alveoli.
D. the oxygen tension of blood in the pulmonary vein is about 5.3 KPa (about 40 mmHg).
E. inspiration is brought about by relaxation of the intercostal muscles.

50. Lung function in normal pregnancy

A. vital capacity is increased by 50%.
B. tidal volume is increased.
C. the subcostal angle is increased.
D. residual volume is reduced.
E. the respiratory rate is decreased.

Index

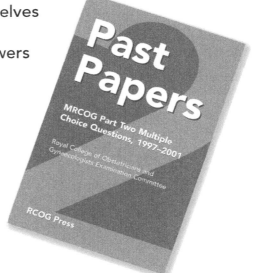

Lightning Source UK Ltd.
Milton Keynes UK
UKOW06f1620120614

233288UK00012B/92/P